# Goodbye To Gout

## A NEW GOUT DIET

by

Rose Scott

### The Truth About What Really Causes Gout.

What To Eat, What Not To Eat & How To Live

An Active Gout Free Life

ISBN - 978-1-9996248-1-1

Published by Roscott Books 2018

DISCLAMER
This book provides general information only. It is based on information gathered from a large number of different sources. It does not provide any form of medical advice and it is not a substitute for the advice of your own doctor, medical practitioner or health care professional. Readers are specifically advised to consult their doctor regarding the treatment of any medical condition that they have. The author of this book shall not be held liable or responsible for any misuse or misunderstanding of the information contained in this book or for any loss, damage or injury caused or alleged to be caused either directly or indirectly by any action that is consequential to reading the contents of this book. No part of this book has been evaluated or approved by any medical, scientific, professional or Food or Drug Administration Authority.

# Contents

# FOREWARD

Suffering from gout is a singularly unpleasant experience, an experience most of us resign ourselves to suffering from for the rest of our lives. Gout adversely affected every part of our life, in fact it had taken over our life. My gout had become so bad that tophi was erupting from one of my big toes. Walking was excruciatingly painful, sleep was impossible, I was unable to work, my life and the life of everyone else in the family was utterly miserable. Then something amazing happened. My wife decided that it was time to see if we could put an end to the pain and distress by finding out what was causing my gout. If we could eliminate the cause then maybe we could eliminate the gout.

Well eliminate it we did. As children of the sixties we had always believed that you are what you eat, so the first place to look was our diet. The challenge was to find out if something we were eating could be causing the gout. Rose researched deep into areas that were initially entirely foreign to her and she tackled complex scientific areas. The more she read the more she realised that there was more to gout than just food, there were certainly no quick fix cures or silver bullets. We made some changes to what we were eating and drinking and we also made some changes to the way we cooked our food. Within weeks the tophi stopped oozing out and the gout flares and swelling in my feet and ankles went away.

When Rose started this work she knew nothing about gout. She had no medical or scientific background either but this proved to be of benefit as it meant that she had no preconceived ideas and was able to 'think outside the box' and challenge the conventional view of what causes gout. The result is a breakthrough in our understanding of gout.

The knowledge we gained from her work was key to us being able to eliminate my gout. There is a light at the end of the tunnel. You really can cure gout if, like us, you use this knowledge as an enabling tool to take control of your life. Rose has turned what we discovered into words that the non scientist can understand and written our story as this comprehensive self help guide. Please read, learn, enjoy and like me make your pulsating swollen red joints a thing of the past.

Jo Scott

# PREFACE

For ten years my husband endured the pain and misery of gout. Five years ago he had reached the end of the road. Gout was destroying our lives. In horrendous pain he was told by an orthopaedic surgeon,

> " *You're eating too many purines and not drinking enough water ..........You're 'crispy'* "

The not drinking enough water we could handle, but what were purines? Neither of us had heard of them. How could something you eat cause such a painful, debilitating disease?

For years I had stood by unable to help so I set myself the task of finding out what purines were and, if they did cause gout, whether eliminating them from our diet would cure it. Little did I know that trying to find the answer to what at the time appeared to be a simple question would be a lifelong change in our diet and this book. With no medical background it was going to be hard work. Like a modern day Miss Marple I set about looking for real scientific evidence, not the old wives' tales and folklore that have shrouded gout for years. What I discovered shocked me. Misinformation - yes, and lots of it, outright lies - possibly, numerous quick fix cures that would never work and a focus on purine rich food that was not supported by scientific evidence.

Does something we eat really cause gout? Well you may be surprised to learn that it does, but the purine rich foods that have hitherto received such a bad press are actually innocent by-standers, the real culprits are some of the things that many of us eat and drink every day of our lives. Move to a gout friendly way of eating and gout goes away, and it goes away for good. It's as simple as that.

Goodbye To Gout is a book that dispels the myths and reveals the truth about what really causes gout. While there are some things you should avoid eating, there are plenty of other things that you can eat and you will be delighted to hear that foods that are high in purines are all firmly back on the menu. With the Goodbye To Gout diet there are no 'forbidden foods', there is no calorie counting and no need for recipes. Instead there is a set of easy to follow guidelines, as opposed to a set of strict rules, that will help you make the switch from the foods that can cause gout to the gout friendly foods that will restore your body's natural balance and set you on the road to being gout free. The occasional mishap will not spell doom. It is what you do most of the time, not what you do some of the time that matters and, unlike some rigidly restricted gout diets, it does not take the fun out of eating.

How many of you would like to be able to say '*I used to have gout*'? Well my husband can. We changed our diet and he now lives an active gout free life. For him, facing a lifetime of pain and medication is a thing of the past.

CHAPTER 1

# Gout - The Disease of Kings

QUESTION: "*What's up with Grand Dad?*"
ANSWER: "*Oh, little Johnny LOOKED at his big toe*"

Well, anyone who suffers from gout or who lives with someone who suffers from gout understands this only too well. The pain is excruciating and even the draught from an open door or the movement of a sheet over a swollen and inflamed big toe or ankle is unbearable. For many, the prospect of living the rest of their life with repeated attacks of gout leaves them in utter despair and for some it can lead to profound depression. Gout is both physically and emotionally debilitating. It takes over your life.

Throughout history gout has been portrayed in a less than flattering light and linked to a life of excess and self indulgence. For centuries it has been the object of satire, often associated with the higher social classes and the copious consumption of rich food. How often have we seen old cartoons of a grotesquely overweight red faced country squire reclining with his wig askew, one foot up on a stool, a glass of wine in his hand and a pipe in the other. Words like gluttony, over indulgence and obesity are all too often used when describing the typical gout patient. Even today gout has a strange sort of blame culture associated with it. The patient is made to feel that in some way he or she is to blame, that it is their own fault that they suffer from the disease and that they have brought it on them self by their own excesses. More often than not this is far from the truth.

## Gout Through The Ages

Gout has afflicted mankind for thousands of years. Egyptian mummies reveal evidence that goes back over 4,000 years and as early as 2600BC it had been identified as a 'disease' by the Egyptians. By the 5th Century BC it was well described by Hippocratic writers who called it the 'un-walkable disease'. It was later nick named Podogra or 'foot pain' because it affects the big toe more than any other part of the body. Gout was extensively studied by the Roman physician Galen (A.D. 131-200) and both Plato and Seneca documented its occurrence and its possible link to diet. Arthritic conditions in skeletal remains of early Pacific islanders and even Neanderthal Man have led paleopathologists to speculate that man's affliction with gout goes back even further.

The prevalence of gout in the ancient world is unknown. In the Middle Ages gout was labelled "*The Disease of Kings*", a disease that only afflicted the rich and the elite and as a consequence only a small minority of the population of the then known world. With the coming of the industrial revolution, increasing urbanisation, changes in living conditions and as a consequence changes also in eating habits, things began to change. But they changed slowly. It is only in the last sixty to seventy years that the incidence of gout has increased significantly and affected a far wider range of people. It is estimated that since the early 1970's the incidence of gout has increased four fold. Over the last twenty years it has more than doubled.

In what is loosely described as the 'Western World', between 1% and 2% of men in their 50's and up to 7% of men in their 70's now suffer from gout. While hither too it was mainly a male disease women, particularly post menopausal women, are now being increasingly afflicted. Why is gout increasing so rapidly? Possible explanations include lifestyle, high levels of pollution, the overall ageing of the population and changes to our diet made possible by increased prosperity and new food manufacturing processes. In reality we just do not know.

## CHAPTER 2

# "You Are What You Eat"

An interesting adage that many people believe to be true. But have you ever wondered where it came from? The origin of the phrase is attributed to the early 19th Century French epicure and gastronome, Anthelme Brillat-Savarin in his book *"Physiologie du Gout"*. A book by the way that had nothing to do with gout, translated it means 'The physiology of Taste'.

In the 1920's and early 30's the nutritionist Victor Lindlahr, who was a strong believer in the idea that the food we eat controls our health, developed the Catabolic Diet. At the time this diet and his views gained some adherents and this led to the earliest known printed example of the saying in an advertisement in the Bridgeport Telegraph in 1923:

*"Ninety per cent of the diseases known to man are caused by cheap food stuffs. You are what you eat"*

Ironically this advertisement was for beef, a food that is widely implicated as being one of the causes of gout. In 1942 Lindlahr published "*You are what you eat; How to win and keep health with diet*" This book appears to be what brought the saying into public awareness. In the 1960's the saying had a new lease of life when the Hippy culture used it as their slogan for healthy eating.

For centuries gout has been linked to diet but when it comes to gout are we really what we eat? Is it possible that diet alone can cause gout? In horrendous pain and with tophi oozing from one of his big toes, my husband was told by an orthopaedic surgeon,

*" You're eating too many purines and not drinking enough water. You're 'crispy' "*

*What's a purine? ... Something you eat, it's in your food"*

Being children of the sixties we had always believed that 'you are what you eat'. In fact we thought our diet was quite healthy, so the challenge was to find out how something we were eating could result in so much pain and distress. Having never heard of the word 'purine' the first thing I did when we got home was to log onto the internet and type in 'what is a purine?' Little did I know then that the end result of this seemingly simple enquiry would be a lifelong change in our diet and this book.

What at first sight looked like finding a simple answer to a simple question left me utterly confused. I kept coming up with words, phrases and terminology that I knew nothing about. I had to keep looking things up on the net. The New Oxford Dictionary never left my side. One question led to another and in the process of answering each question my learning curve became immense. My knowledge of biochemistry and human physiology just grew and grew. In order to understand everything I was reading it had to. So forty years on I was effectively back in the class room learning about subjects that were not on the curriculum or didn't even exist when I was at school. This proved to be a time consuming process as I was going two steps forward and then one step back, constantly looking up words, acronyms, technical terms and topics. The end result was a 'glossary', which is included at the end of this book and a series of 'primers' or short lessons on some of the topics that I needed to understand before I could move forward. Primers on:-

1. Organic and Inorganic Compounds
2. Metabolism, Enzymes and Co-Factors
3. Carbohydrates, Proteins and Amino Acids
4. Fats, Lipids and Polyunsaturated Fatty Acids
5. Vitamins and Minerals
6. Insulin, Leptin and Ghrelin
7. Metabolic Syndrome
8. Glycemic Index
9. Saturated Solutions and Crystallisation
10. pH and Acidosis
11. The Redox Cycle
12. Free Radicals and Antioxidants
13. Oxidative Stress
14. Inflammation
15. How Purines Become Uric Acid

are included in the Appendix. Without this knowledge I was going no where so, if like me, you need to update yourself on any of these topics, go to the Appendix before you read on.

So if its true that "you are what you eat", what should the gout sufferer be eating; which foods are good to eat, which foods are not so good and which foods are just plain bad? For years science and the medical profession have told us that purines cause gout and that a low purine diet will cure it. If you log onto the Internet there are many sites and even 'learned journals' still telling you the same thing. But is this really true? For me purines and a low purine diet did not make sense. As long ago as 1984 a scientist called Irvine Fox who studied gout in great detail noted that a low purine diet was ineffective and had only a minor effect on gout. In reality a low purine diet is well nigh impossible to follow and it is probably one of the worse possible diets for gout simply because it is so imbalanced.

As I studied and read more, purines began to look more and more like innocent bye standers. The guilty party appeared to be not just one thing. It was more likely to be a combination of not only food but also lifestyle and possibly even the cooking methods that have found their way into the western diet and western culture over the last sixty to seventy years.

CHAPTER 3

# The Causes of Gout

Gout is the most common form of inflammatory arthritis found in industrialised countries. It affects between 1% and 2% of adult men in their 50's and up to 7% of men in their 70's. The most recent research in the UK used the Clinical Research Data Link to analyse existing and new cases of gout between 1997 and 2012. Of the 4.5 million eligible candidates on the database 116,000 already had gout and 7,000 new cases were identified during the course of the study. Within this group the prevalence of gout rose by 64% during the 15 years over which the study was undertaken, an astonishing increase of around 4% a year.

Of all of the forms of arthritis gout is the one we understand the best, yet despite this the actual "cause" of gout still remains somewhat obscure. Over the years medical science has studied it in great detail and correlated its occurrence to both diet and lifestyle. In the process it has gained a good understanding of how it affects the body, but with the development of Allopurinol and other drugs such as Probenecid interest in finding out what actually causes gout diminished. Gout became a 'treatable' disease and, as is so often the case, the 'cure' became more important than understanding the cause and preventing the onset of the disease in the first place. However, as the treatment of gout is often poorly managed and only around 40% of the medications prescribed are actually effective, there is still a real need to understand more about the disease. Only by understanding the cause can we find out what we need to do to prevent the disease developing in the first place, and once it has developed, hopefully halt its progress, turn back the clock and stop it.

What we do know is that gout is all to do with uric acid, a weak organic acid that occurs naturally in your blood, and the monosodium urate crystals that it sometimes forms. If you suffer from gout you are likely to have a higher than 'normal' amount of uric acid in your blood (in medical terms you suffer from hyperuricemia) and, because uric acid is not very soluble, monosodium urate crystals have formed and accumulated in the soft tissue in one or some of your joints. Most commonly a big toe or an ankle is the target but any joint can be affected. Your body sees these crystals as 'foreign bodies' and your immune system responds accordingly, sending out antibodies to fight them off. Hence the inflammation and from this the excruciating pain.

But, did you know that not everyone with a high level of uric acid will develop gout? In fact only between 10% - 20% of individuals with 'hyperuricemia' will actually develop gout. What is known for sure is that for most people, once monosodium urate crystals have formed, gout 'flares' or attacks will recur over and over again, usually at increasingly frequent intervals.

Men naturally have higher levels of uric acid than women and as a consequence an increased prevalence of gout. This however becomes less pronounced as we get older. Why the difference between men and women? Well it may be explained in women of childbearing age by the presence of oestrogen, which is known to have the effect of making the kidneys more efficient at removing uric acid. As a consequence gout is rare in young women. However, post menopause as oestrogen levels fall, uric acid levels increase and gout becomes more prevalent. By the time they reach their 70's women are just as likely to develop gout as men.

It seems very strange that something that causes so much trouble and such intense pain should exist in the human body at all. Before we go any further at trying to understand hyperuricemia, the fundamental cause of gout, and why only one in five of the people who suffer from it develop gout, we need to understand where uric acid comes from.

CHAPTER 4

# Uric Acid & Purines

Uric acid is formed inside our bodies when purines are broken down or 'catabolised'. Because of this purines are often said to be the bane of the gout sufferers life and for years we have been told to avoid them or to reduce their intake. Because of their association with gout purines have acquired a reputation of being in some way 'bad'. Yet nothing could be farther from the truth.

Purines are one of two groups of molecules that contain nitrogen. In biochemical terms they are called 'nitrogenous bases. The other family of nitrogenous bases are Pyrimidines. In the natural living world purines and pyrimidines are found everywhere and some scientists believe that they existed on earth before life as we know it began. The isolation of purines from meteorites that were formed when our solar system was born provides evidence that these molecules could also be present in other solar systems.

Purines and pyrimidines are found in all of the living organisms on earth, from simple viruses to complex multi-cellular creatures. Because they provide some of the chemical structures of both DNA (Deoxyribonucleic acid), and RNA (Ribonucleic acid), they are in pretty much every cell of plants, animals and humans alike. As such they are among the most important of all biological molecules on earth. Without these nitrogenous bases our chromosomes, and the genetic material in all living creatures including viruses and bacteria, would not exist. Living cells could not produce energy or make many of the molecules they need to function.

DNA and RNA are made from the two 'nitrogenous bases', the purines, ( Adenine and Guanine ), and the pyrimidines, (Thymine, Cytosine, and Uracil ). In using these nature has been incredibly economical as these two groups of nitrogenous bases are all that is needed to produce the amazing diversity of species that live on planet earth. When one purine base is paired with one pyrimidine base, a 'base pair' is formed. When base pairs are joined together to form double-stranded, ladder-like chains of DNA, and when the DNA is coiled into chromosomes, the billions of base pairs that constitute the human genome can be stored within the nucleus of each of our cells and, in the same way, the cells of all other living things on earth.

When cells are broken down, either when they are consumed as food or they die as a result of an organisms natural programmed cell death, a process called Apoptosis, the purines in the cells are metabolised. How they are metabolised is fascinating. Lower species such as microbes process the purines to the end product of ammonia. However, as you progress up the evolutionary ladder the breakdown and metabolism of the purines becomes less and less complete. At the top of the evolutionary ladder, in humans and the higher primates, uric acid is one of the end products, but in other mammals something different happens. This is because the majority of mammals have an enzyme called Uricase which continues the breakdown or 'catabolism' of the purines by converting the uric acid into a substance called Allantoin. Unlike uric acid Allantoin is a very soluble substance that dissolves easily and is freely excreted in their urine.

So why the difference between humans, the higher primates and other mammals? Many millions of years ago the apes and higher primates that were to become the early hominids had the same active uricase gene as all of the other mammals. However, about 26 million years ago in the Miocene Epoch a series of mutations of the uricase gene began and within 13 million years the gene had completely lost its functionality. The early humans and the higher primates no longer had the ability to break down purines to allantoin, the process ended with uric acid. The biological reasons for the loss of activity of the uricase gene are not known. While there are many theories and a lot of speculation about it, there is no doubt that these mutations and the existence of uric acid must have given our early ancestors an important evolutionary advantage.

## What is Uric Acid?

What is its purpose? Is it "good" or is it "bad"?

For many years uric acid was considered to be an inert waste product that, when present in higher than normal levels, was known for the harmful and troublesome effects of causing gout and kidney stones. Even now many sources of information on gout tell you that *"uric acid serves no biochemical function"*. However, we now know much more about uric acid's various biochemical functions and its beneficial effects and one of these is that it is a powerful antioxidant. In fact uric acid has the highest concentration of any of the water soluble antioxidants found in our blood and it provides nearly half of the antioxidant capacity that our blood contains. Its antioxidant properties are fifty times as powerful as those of Vitamin C, an antioxidant that most of us have heard of.

## Why does our body need antioxidants?

The majority of life forms on earth need oxygen to live. One of the strange things about this is that oxygen exists as a highly reactive molecule that can damage living organisms by producing free radicals. Heard of free radicals but don't really know what they are? Well a few years ago that was me. Put simply, a free radical is an atom, molecule or ion that is 'unstable'. This instability is due to the atomic or molecular structure of the free radical. Any molecule or atom that has one or more unpaired electrons in its outer orbit is known as a free radical. Another term that is sometimes used to describe free radicals is Reactive Oxygen Species or ROS. Because they are unstable, free radicals attempt to stabilise themselves by 'stealing' electrons from other atoms, molecules or ions.

Free radicals are all around us. The UV rays from the sun create them when we are exposed to sunlight, we breath them in, especially from polluted air, and we consume them in our food. Simply by living our bodies produce free radicals. Some of these are needed in controlled amounts to keep us healthy. Our immune system depends heavily on them. However, some of the free radicals we are exposed to can cause damage, sometimes severe damage, and these free radicals need to be neutralised and rendered harmless. In order to do this we need antioxidants. When there is an imbalance between free radicals and the body's ability to render them harmless or repair the damage they have caused a state of 'oxidative stress' results. When this happens cells, proteins and DNA can become damaged. Severe oxidative stress can have toxic effects that can result in widespread cell death and ultimately disease. In animal studies investigating diseases caused by oxidative stress, scientists have found that uric acid is able to both prevent the diseases from developing and also, once they have developed, reduce their severity.

The antioxidant properties of uric acid are however complex. It only reacts with some of the free radicals that it finds in our body and sometimes it only works effectively as an antioxidant if Vitamin C is also present. One other function of uric acid that is of particular interest is that as well as working along side Vitamin C, it also protects and conserves the Vitamin C. Because the ions of some of the trace elements our bodies need, such as iron and manganese, are 'unstable' they have the effect of 'binding' to the Vitamin C and as a consequence using it up and making it ineffective as an antioxidant. However, uric acid is able to take the place of the Vitamin C and 'bind' itself to these metals. This has the effect of conserving the Vitamin C, a Vitamin that is essential for our existence. Because of the way uric acid protects Vitamin C some scientists have speculated that the existence of uric acid may be an evolutionary adaptation to our inability to make Vitamin C, a Vitamin that most other animals are able to make for themselves. When the early primates lost their ability to make Vitamin C through a genetic mutation between 40 and 50 million years ago, long before the mutations to the uricase gene, they lived in a sort of perpetual summer and ate large quantities of Vitamin C in a diet that was mainly leaves and fruit. Later on however, as the climate changed and changes in their diet occurred, less Vitamin C from vegetation was available to them, so the lack of the Vitamin C would have been mitigated by the loss of uricase activity and the existence of uric acid.

The scientific community has known about uric acid's function as an antioxidant since 1981. But despite this it is something that is seldom mentioned. When you read about gout, uric acid is invariably depicted as being 'bad', a sort of villain that only causes trouble. This is clearly not the case. Our bodies need uric acid, in fact without it they would simply not function properly. Yet just as there is "good" and "bad" cholesterol, uric acid is also something of a paradox. As an antioxidant it is effectively one of the body's 'champions', protecting it from damage by neutralising the oxidation effect of free radicals. But when it is present in higher than normal amounts or with other essential vitamins or micro nutrients missing, it in fact becomes pro oxidant and pro inflammatory, and as a consequence can itself cause damage.

## When does Uric Acid behave badly?

An interesting example of uric acid behaving badly is when it affects insulin levels and the way our bodies handle the glucose in our blood. Uric acid inhibits and slows down the production of a substance called nitric oxide. Insulin needs nitric oxide to stimulate the uptake of glucose, so with high levels of uric acid and low levels of nitric oxide the insulin in our blood is less able to handle glucose and the level of sugar in our blood increases. In order for the body to cope with the high level of sugar it produces more insulin and slowly insulin resistance develops. Ultimately, over time, this can lead to type two diabetes.

Uric acid is also the subject of an antioxidant and pro-oxidant paradox that is often referred to as the REDOX shuttle. Being an antioxidant, uric acid can react with a number of different free radicals and Reactive Oxygen Species that it finds in our bodies and render them harmless. When this happens it is broken down in stages to form a number of different end products. However, some of these end products are unstable and as a consequence they behave like free radicals. Under balanced conditions these unstable end products can be rendered harmless by the Vitamin C or other antioxidants that are also present and their potential damaging effect is neutralised. However, if there is not enough Vitamin C or other antioxidants around to do this the end result is that what was initially a beneficial antioxidant process is now made into a damaging pro oxidant process and uric acid free radicals are created.

So the answer to the question, *Is uric acid good or is it bad?* is that when it is good it is very good but on some occasions, and in circumstances that appear to depend on where it is in the body and what other biochemicals are around at the same time, it can also be very bad.

The relationship between uric acid and the human body is complex and many questions about the part it plays have yet to be answered. One thing is certain however, the human body needs uric acid. It is an essential part of our body's biochemistry and it plays a major role in its antioxidant defences. Is uric acid the only antioxidant our body makes? No. It is just one of a sophisticated team of antioxidants and enzymes that behave like antioxidants that our bodies make in order to protect itself from free radicals and repair any oxidative damage that free radicals have caused. Superoxide Dismutase (SOD), Glutathione Peroxidase (GPX), Alpha Lipoic acid (ALA), Catalase and Coenzyme Q10 (CoQ10) are just some of our endogenous antioxidants that all work together as part of this team; some have specialised roles in terms of which free radicals they are most effective against, some are water soluble, some are fat soluble and some only work in specific parts of our bodies. Superoxide Dismutase and Glutathione are particularly important antioxidants as our body appears to be able to more or less 'make them to order' when certain types of free radicals are present.

## Where Do the Purines Come From?

Well, food is one source of purines but our own bodies also provide a source of purines when our cells die, either through the natural process of 'programmed' cell death or Apoptosis, or because cells become damaged by free radicals and other damage causing agents. The amount of purine coming from our own body is surprisingly high. Some scientists say that 70% of the purines our body uses come from ourselves (endogenous purines) and 30% from our food ( exogenous purines ), others that up to 90% come from our bodies and only 10% from our food. Clearly if the body is under stress and cells die or become damaged and need to be replaced in higher than normal numbers the ratio between the purines we eat and the purines our bodies produce will change.

## How are the purines converted into uric acid?

The interaction between purines and body chemistry is complicated. Understanding the purine and uric acid connection is far from straightforward, particularly for a 'lay person' with limited scientific knowledge. It took me quite a while to begin to understand it. As with all metabolic and catabolic processes, enzymes are needed and in the case of uric acid the last one in a long multi stage process is the enzyme Xanthine Oxidase. If you have too little Xanthine Oxidase you don't make enough uric acid and if you have too much you have the potential to make too much uric acid. The drug Allopurinol that is used to treat gout inhibits the way Xanthine Oxidase works and as a consequence it reduces the amount of uric acid the body is able to produce.

Irrespective of whether they come from the food we eat or from our own bodies the two purine 'bases' Guanine and Adenine are the compounds that break down and ultimately form uric acid. None of the three pyrimidines are involved in the process. For completeness the breakdown of purines into uric acid has been included in the Primer section, *'How purines become uric acid'*.

The breakdown of purines and their conversion into uric acid is a major biological source of free radicals that are produced in the form of 'superoxide'. Under normal healthy balanced conditions these superoxides are rendered harmless by one of the body's own antioxidants, Superoxide Dismutase (SOD). However, if conditions are not balanced and for some reason the body is unable to supply enough Superoxide Dismutase, the excess superoxide generated acts as a free radical and ultimately ends up contributing to and increasing the state of oxidative stress in the body. This in turn leads to the influx of inflammatory cells and general state of inflammation that can trigger the onset of many chronic diseases.

So where does inflammation fit into the picture?

CHAPTER 5

# Inflammation & Our Immune System

Inflammation is a topic that is attracting a lot of attention at the moment as it appears to be associated with many of the chronic diseases that are afflicting the Western World. Gout is a form of inflammatory arthritis, so if you have gout parts of your body are in a state of inflammation. Because of this understanding inflammation and how it affects your body is important.

The word inflammation comes from the Latin word '*inflammo*' meaning '*I set alight, I ignite*'. When something harmful or irritating affects a part of your body there is an automatic response to try to remove it. When you catch a cold or sprain your ankle your immune system moves into gear and triggers a chain of events that is referred to as the inflammatory cascade. The familiar signs of inflammation, raised temperature, localised heat, pain, swelling and redness, are the first signs that your immune system is being called into action and they show you that your body is trying to heal itself.

Inflammation is part of the body's 'innate' immune response, something that is present even before we are born. Innate immunity is an automatic immunity that is not directed towards anything specific. As we go through life and are exposed to diseases or vaccinated against them we acquire 'adaptive' immunity. In a delicate balance of give-and-take inflammation begins when 'pro-inflammatory hormones' in your body call out for your white blood cells to come and clear out an infection or repair damaged tissue. These pro-inflammatory hormones are matched by equally powerful closely related 'anti-inflammatory' compounds which move in once the threat is neutralised to begin the healing process.

The inflammation we experience during our daily lives can be either 'acute' or 'chronic'. Chronic inflammation is sometimes referred to as 'systemic' inflammation. Acute inflammation that ebbs and flows as needed signifies a well balanced immune system. Colds, flu and childhood diseases mean that inflammation and a rise in temperature starts suddenly and quickly progresses to become severe. The signs and symptoms are only present for a few days and they soon subside. On occasion in cases of severe illness they can last for a few weeks but this is unusual.

Sometimes, however, as in the case of chronic or systemic inflammation, the inflammation itself can cause further inflammation. It can become self perpetuating and sometimes last for months or even years. Symptoms of inflammation that do not go away are telling you that the switch to your immune system is stuck in the 'on' position. It is poised on high alert and is unable to shut itself off. Some people believe that chronic irritants, food sensitivities and common allergens like proteins found in dairy products and wheat can trigger this type of chronic inflammation. It is now a widely accepted fact that the food we eat can be either 'pro' or 'anti' inflammatory.

The study of inflammation and our immune system is a relatively new science. While there is still an enormous amount to learn there is no doubt that the human immune response is an extremely sophisticated finely balanced mechanism. Without it we would not be able to survive the most minor infection or the tiniest cut. Some scientists believe that like other things in our evolutionary history this sophisticated immune response gave our early ancestors a major survival advantage. As with so much about the human body how such a sophisticated response came about is unclear. It is certainly the subject of a great deal of speculation. However, some believe that evolution may have had yet another incentive for losing the uricase gene and giving us uric acid.

Inflammation occurs when tissues in our body are damaged or when we are 'attacked' by bacteria or viruses. Substances like pro inflammatory hormones are produced by our body and these alert it to the danger and tell our immune system to switch itself on. Uric acid behaves like one of these pro inflammatory hormones. It is not involved in our immune response to bacteria and viruses but it is involved when our bodies are subjected to trauma and cells are damaged or die. The large amounts of uric acid that are produced in the immediate vicinity of damaged, dying or dead cells stimulates a type of immune cell called dendritic cells to mature and swing into action. Effectively uric acid has a sort of immune boosting effect and it plays a fundamental part in protecting our bodies from tissue damage and trauma. If this theory is correct, by lacking the ability to breakdown and degrade purines to the soluble form of allantoin, uric acid came to the rescue of the higher primates and enabled them to develop a robust defence against injury and large scale tissue damage. This would have given them a substantial survival advantage.

In the Western World chronic or systemic inflammation is on the rise. We know this from inflammatory markers and the pro inflammatory and anti inflammatory hormones that our body's produce. Most degenerative diseases involve an element of chronic low level inflammation and the inability to turn off important inflammatory processes when they are no longer needed. Gout is one of these diseases.

CHAPTER 6

# Crystals of Uric Acid

Before we try to answer the question of what causes uric acid levels to rise, we first need to understand what makes uric acid crystals form and why only between 10% and 20% of the people with high levels of uric acid go on to develop gout.

In people who suffer from gout crystals of uric acid accumulate in the form of Tophi, usually within a joint. Sometimes these Tophi are close to the surface of the skin and appear as white or yellowish white nodules. In severe cases of advanced gout these Tophi can burst open and release a creamy white substance. In 1679 a scientist called Leeuwenhoek was the first person to observe and describe 'crystals' in gouty tophus. These were later identified as being crystals of uric acid in 1797. For over 150 years uric acid crystals were known to be the cause of gout but they were only actually seen in detail in a polarising microscope in 1961.

In humans the 'normal' concentration of uric acid that is commonly found today is fairly close to the point at which crystals will form. At the normal body temperature of 37 deg C, once uric acid levels reach between 6.8 and 7.0mg/dl monosodium urate crystals can begin to form. The more uric acid there is in the blood the more likely it is that crystals will form and accumulate in joints. When uric acid levels are lower than 6mg/dl i.e. below saturation point, in the absence of a gout flare, no new crystals will form and existing crystals will slowly dissolve, ultimately preventing further acute gout flares and joint damage. The lower the uric acid level the faster the monosodium urate crystals will dissolve. There is good evidence that uric acid levels below 6mg/dl will result in gradual freedom from gout attacks and that concentrations lower than 5mg/dl will ultimately lead to the shrinkage and eventual disappearance of Tophi. There is also some evidence to suggest that the lower the level of uric acid level is the faster the Tophi will reduce in size.

Levels of uric acid that are described as 'normal' can be anywhere in the range 3mg/dl to 7mg/dl. With such a wide range what is 'high' for one person is 'normal' for another. Hyperuricemia is not a 'disease' as such but more an underlying factor that predisposes someone towards developing gout. It does not automatically cause it. We are told over and over again that if you have hyperuricemia you will develop gout, but we know that only between 10% and 20% of people with hyperuricemia will actually develop it. In a benchmark study over a five year period, 22% of the men who had uric acid levels higher than 9mg/dl developed gout, a much higher rate than men with uric acid levels lower than 9mg/dl. Nevertheless, this means that 78% of the men who had uric acid levels above 9mg/d did not develop gout during the five year period of the study. We therefore have to ask ourselves what other factors, when combined with high levels of uric acid, make crystals form and trigger the first attack of gout.

Sustained high levels of uric acid will eventually lead to what is effectively a super saturated solution of uric acid in the blood, but before the monosodium urate crystals form a 'crystallisation event' needs to take place. Monosodium urate crystals are very small and very fragile so once they have formed in joints they fracture easily into tiny fragments and these small fragments then 'seed' new crystals that can grow very quickly. Research has made substantial progress in understanding how crystals behave once they are formed, but the underlying mechanisms that initiate the first transition event from super saturated solution to crystal is still not fully understood.

Typically, uric acid levels higher than 6.8 mg/dl are defined as hyperuricemia. However, crystallization at this concentration at normal body temperature is very difficult to reproduce in the laboratory. Also, gout attacks tend to have a rapid onset, whereas the crystallization process in the laboratory is quite slow. So what other factors, when combined with high levels of uric acid, contribute to the formation of crystals? The simple answer to this is that rather than one specific cause, there are believed to be several possible causes that combine together to give rise to a sort of 'catastrophe situation' in which the first crystals form:-

- Under laboratory conditions we know that irritation and minor physical trauma or even mechanical shock, such as breaking a laboratory slide, will cause crystals to form in a saturated solution of uric acid. We also know that crystals are more likely to form at lower temperatures. At between 32 and 33 deg C crystals can form with uric acid concentrations as low as 3mg/dl. This is interesting as with gout, uric acid crystals usually form in extremes of the body such as toes, fingers, elbows and ears, where the body temperature is lower than normal and can often be as low as 32 deg C.

- The concentration of uric acid can be 100 times higher in the fluid found around damaged and dying cells than in the blood, so damaged or dying cells create a local micro environment of a highly super saturated solution in which uric acid crystals can form. We know that the large-scale cell death resulting from the chemotherapy and radiation therapy used to treat cancer often induces the precipitation of Monosodium Urate crystals, and as a consequence uric acid levels are actively managed as part of chemotherapy and radiation therapy in order to avoid the onset of an attack of gout in an otherwise gout free patient.

- In order for any crystal to form or 'nucleate' it needs a microscopic particle or 'seed' around which to grow. Under laboratory conditions nucleation is significantly enhanced when calcium ions are present. There are two things that could increase the concentration of calcium ions:-

1: It is known that the concentration of calcium ions in the blood increases rapidly with acidosis, i.e. if the pH of the blood falls to below its 'normal' level. So any factor that lowers the pH of the blood could increase the chance of a crystal forming around a calcium ion. This is where things start to get a bit complicated. In order for our body and its cells to work properly the pH of our blood needs to be in the range 7.35 to 7.45. When we eat food and drink liquids the end products of their digestion can have an acid or alkaline effect on our blood. In addition, as our cells produce energy and simply 'live' a number of different acids are formed. Because it is essential that the pH of our blood is kept between 7.35 and 7.45 the body has three major 'buffering' mechanisms that it uses to keep the pH within this range. One of these is the phosphate buffer system and this uses different phosphate ions in our body to neutralise acids. About 85% of these come from calcium phosphate salts which are components of our bones and teeth. If our body is regularly exposed to large amounts of acid forming foods and drink over a long period of time our phosphate buffer can run low so the body draws on its calcium phosphate reserves, taking small amounts of it from our bones and teeth. The end result is the increased concentration of calcium ions in the blood and the increased risk of monosodium urate crystals forming around them.

2: Our bodies contain a natural substances known as 'sulphated mucopolysaccharides'. These 'glue' cells together and form part of the connective tissue that lubricates our joints. These 'sulphated mucopolysaccharides' are known to diminish and break down as we get older. They are also known to hold large amounts of calcium and it has been suggested that their breakdown could result in the release of calcium and an increase in the local concentrations of calcium ions in exactly the place where monosodium urate crystals will form, in the connective tissue of joints. One of these mucopolysaccharides, mitochondria sulphate, is made in our bodies from glucosamine but its synthesis can be inhibited by nutritional deficiencies in vitamins and minerals such as Vitamin C, Manganese and Vitamin A . Anti inflammatory drugs, stress, trauma and dehydration can all have an adverse effect on the way mitochondria sulphate is made by our bodies.

- One final thing that is often overlooked, is that gout attacks usually begin during the night when we are asleep. This was first observed in 1683 by Dr Thomas Sydenham who wrote about it in great detail. We now understand why this happens. Sleep apnoea is a relatively common disorder that causes interrupted breathing and shallow infrequent breathing during sleep. Like extreme exercise, the consumption of large amounts of alcohol and fasting, sleep apnoea can lead to a sudden increase in the amount of lactic acid in our blood. This has not only the effect of reducing the amount of uric acid that the body excretes, it also creates a sudden, short-term, acidic 'spike' in the pH of the blood that can increase the number of calcium ions present and hence seed the formation of crystals.

What we have is a complex picture that suggests a number of possible reasons why the first crystals of uric acid form; trauma from an accidental blow, large scale cell death or damage from free radicals that have overwhelmed our body's antioxidant defences or an increase in the concentration of calcium ions due to a metabolic upset or a sudden change in pH that could be due to extreme exercise, sleep apnoea or the over consumption of alcohol. However, once crystals have formed the first gout attack will follow. The body's innate immune response quickly detects the newly appearing uric acid crystals and assumes that they are diseased or damaged cells. In response white blood cells are sent to attack the 'invaders', but when they try to devour them the uric acid crystals burst the cells and as the white blood cells die, they release proteins telling the immune system that the cell has lost its fight with the invader and that reinforcements need to be sent in. The released proteins also generate lactic acid and this lowers the pH of the blood. As noted above, in order to bring the pH back to normal the body's phosphate buffering system swings into action, so increasing the concentration of calcium ions which causes more crystals to form. The immune system responds by sending in more white blood cells. More white blood cells are killed by the uric acid crystals causing even more proteins and lactic acid to be released and more crystals to form. This process perpetuates itself creating a runaway inflammatory response and the extreme pain of gout.

In the end the process is self limiting because the concentration of uric acid reduces as it is consumed by the growing crystals and the pH level of the blood returns to normal. This explains the fact that uric acid levels often reduce during gout attacks, sometimes to within normal ranges. However, after the gout flare has subsided you are left with what is effectively a permanent low grade systemic inflammation with increased levels of C- Reactive Protein and inflammatory cytokines and a body that in immunological terms is 'sensitised' to uric acid crystals and in a state of high alert, waiting for the next attack.

CHAPTER 7

# What Is Hyperuricemia?

Hyperuricemia has on occasion been described as being a plague of the western world and it is thought by some to be the cause of many of the chronic diseases that are increasing so rapidly. However, there are others who believe that there is no evidence to support this. They believe that hyperuricemia is either a risk factor for these diseases or the result of them but not the cause. Whatever the case may be, there is a clear link between hyperuricemia and metabolic syndrome, the precursor of many of these chronic diseases. Metabolic syndrome is thought to affect 1 in 4 adults in the UK and up to 1 in 3 adults in the United States. Not heard of metabolic syndrome? Well, it is a term used to describe a combination of insulin resistance, poor glucose tolerance, high blood pressure, high levels of bad cholesterol and low levels of good cholesterol (dyslipidemia), certain kidney conditions and above normal BMI (body mass index) or the 'accumulation of visceral fat'. It puts you at increased risk of heart disease, stroke and other conditions affecting blood vessels.

The prevalence of metabolic syndrome increases substantially with increasing levels of uric acid, from 19% when uric acid levels are below 6mg/dl to 91% when uric acid levels are 10mg.dl or higher. Is there a link between metabolic syndrome and gout? Well the most recent studies in America show that there is. In a representative sample of adult men and women with gout 63% of them also had metabolic syndrome, compared to 25% in individuals without gout. In other words, metabolic syndrome is remarkably high in individuals with gout and hyperuricemia.

When it comes to gout hyperuricemia is most certainly a causative factor as it is almost always present when gout develops. Only a few cases of gout in people with levels of uric acid that are below the 'normal' bounds have ever been recorded. It is a very rare event.

So what exactly is Hyperuricemia and what causes uric acid levels to rise? Hyperuricemia is defined as being:-

"... a level of uric acid in the blood that is higher than 'normal'. In humans, for women the upper end of the normal range is 6mg/dl for men it is between 6.5mg/dl - 7.0mg/dl ..."

A normal adult male has a 'pool ' of uric aid in his body of approximately 1200 mg. This is twice the amount of an adult female. Normally, the uric acid measured is assumed to be soluble, so when insoluble crystals of uric acid are deposited, as in gout, the amount of uric acid measured is almost invariably underestimated.

The amount of uric acid in the blood and the incidence of hyperuricemia varies considerably among populations. It can be influenced by many factors, including ethnic background, age, sex and body weight and a variety of drugs and medications can all affect the amount of uric acid.

Since the early half of the 20th Century uric acid levels have risen significantly among Americans. In the 1920s, average uric acid levels were about 3.5 mg/dl. By 1980, average uric acid levels had climbed into the range of 6.0 to 6.5 mg/dl and they are without doubt much higher now. In a study in America, the prevalence of hyperuricemia in people over 75 was shown to have doubled between 1990 and 1999. A similar trend has also been observed in studies in developing countries. Asia, and in particular Taiwan, having the biggest increase.

## Recycling Uric Acid - the body needs it

The regulation of the amount of uric acid we have in our blood is a complex process. The production of uric acid and its excretion are balanced processes in which, under normal circumstances, about two thirds of the uric acid turned over daily is excreted by the kidneys and virtually all of the rest is eliminated by bacteria in the digestive tract. The kidney filters out uric acid but then reclaims some of what it has filtered through 're-uptake' The amount of uric acid that is re-absorbed through re-uptake is surprisingly high. Of the uric acid the kidneys filter out only between 6% and 12% is actually excreted. Such an effort to stop the removal of what was once thought to be a metabolic or biological "waste product" implies that there must be some considerable advantages associated with holding on to uric acid.

Why does the body want to hang onto Uric Acid? Well I'm not sure, and its one of the things I haven't been able to really get to the bottom of. However, uric acid is 'turned over' about every twenty hours and this compares to a turnover or 'life' of only four hours for Vitamin C. This makes uric acid a fairly long lived antioxidant in terms of body chemistry. A possible theory I have for why the body 'recycles' uric acid, and I stress that I have not seen this written down anywhere, is that the body needs iron to make Xanthine Oxidase, one of the enzymes that converts purines into uric acid. So when people have low levels of iron they can be deficient in Xanthine Oxidase and as a consequence only able to make a small amount of uric acid. Low levels of zinc also cause lower levels of uric acid. In a vegetarian diet there is much less iron and zinc available than in a diet that is based on animal protein, and the iron that is available is more difficult for the body to absorb than the HEME iron found in meat. So maybe our bodies evolved to recycle uric acid at a time when we ate a mainly vegetarian diet and as a consequence both iron and zinc were in short supply.

## What causes hyperuricemia & why do uric acid levels rise?

Hyperuricemia is thought to result from either the over production of uric acid, the under excretion of uric acid or a combination of both. It can also be a primary or secondary result of a medical condition or the use of certain types of drugs and medication. Although I have been unable to verify the source of these figures, the general consensus is that the over production of uric acid accounts for 10% of the cases of hyperuricemia and the under excretion of uric acid for 90%.

On the assumption that these figures are correct, before we take a look at the reasons why we produce too much uric acid or fail to excrete enough, it is worth noting that the conventional 'low purine' diet that is recommended for gout does not hold up. A low purine diet addresses the 10% issue of the over production of uric acid, and 70% of the purines for this over production will come from the body's own turnover of cells. Diet therefore would contribute at best only 30% of this 10%, in other words 3%, a very small amount. In view of this logic says that the 'excessive intake of dietary purines' can rarely if ever be the *cause* of the over production of uric acid.

## Why do we produce too much uric acid?

If the over production of uric acid accounts for 10% of the cases of hyperuricemia, why do our bodies produce too much uric acid?

### The Enzyme Xanthine Oxidase:

Xanthine Oxidase is the last enzyme in a chain of enzymes that the body needs to breakdown purines into uric acid. On the assumption that there is a supply of purines available it makes sense that if you have a lot of active Xanthine Oxidase you have the capability of making a lot of uric acid. Conversely if you only have a small amount of Xanthine Oxidase or you lack the building blocks from which it is made, you can only produce a small amount of uric acid. So what stimulates the body to make Xanthine Oxidase and what suppresses it?

Hyperuricemia resulting from too much Xanthine Oxidase activity is treated with the drug Allopurinol. This acts as a Xanthine Oxidase inhibitor and has the effect of reducing the amount of Xanthine Oxidase that is available to transform purines into uric acid. It doesn't address the issue of what is stimulating the production of the uric acid.

One of the little known facts about gout is the link to iron that was mentioned earlier. Because iron in a readily available form is needed to make Xanthine Oxidase, the presence of a lot of iron can stimulate the production of Xanthine Oxidase. In addition, iron binds to and destroys Vitamin C and Vitamin C is something that the body tries very hard to hang on to. As uric acid has the ability to protect the Vitamin C by binding to the iron and rendering it inactive, high levels of iron could be involved in the regulation of uric acid and stimulate its production in an attempt by the body to protect the Vitamin C.

In the light of this, suppressing the activity of Xanthine Oxidase with Allopurinol does not entirely make sense, well at least to the lay person.

To quote from one learned body:-

> "Rather than preventing the generation of uric acid, a remarkably beneficial iron chelator and antioxidant, with Allopurinol or increasing its urinary excretion with Probenecid, perhaps a more rational treatment for hyperuricemia might be not only the avoidance of highly absorbable iron in red meat, but also regular voluntary donations of blood to decrease the relatively elevated body iron stores of men and post menopausal women, thereby balancing decreased uric acid production with antioxidant needs."

Intriguing!! So what else do we know about why we produce too much uric acid?

## Fructose: An important player in Hyperuricemia.

Fructose is a simple sugar, a 'monosaccharide', that is found in fruit and vegetables. Table sugar (sucrose) is a 'disaccharide' sugar that is made from one molecule of fructose and one molecule of glucose. When we metabolise table sugar it breaks down into separate molecules of glucose and fructose. Unlike glucose, fructose does not directly stimulate the production of insulin, so for many years it was thought to be a good type of sugar for people with diabetes to use. Because it does not directly stimulate the production of insulin and the satiety hormone Leptin, it a has the effect of increasing the concentration of the hunger hormone Ghrelin and this leads to us eating more and consuming more calories than we need. Ultimately we gain weight.

Like all sugars Fructose is a carbohydrate. However, it is the only carbohydrate known to directly increase the amount of uric acid in the blood. 'Fructose induced hyperuricemia' has been know about for some time. It was first reported in The Lancet in the 1960's and further research in the 1980's confirmed the previous research and identified the mechanisms through which hyperuricemia could be induced by fructose. A review of available literature that was published in 1993 concluded that in healthy individuals, diets that were high in fructose were likely to give rise to hyperuricemia.

Contrary to what we are sometimes led to believe, fructose is not an alien substance and it is not a 'poison'. When it is consumed in naturally occurring amounts as part of a natural 'whole' food it is relatively benign. For instance when we eat an apple or an orange. However, when it is consumed in a 'pure' unnatural form or in large amounts it can have an extremely damaging effect on the body. Unlike glucose, which is used as a source of energy throughout our body, fructose does not provide us directly with a source of energy. It is processed primarily in the liver and converted into glycogen. If you consume a lot of fructose in the easily digested form found in soft drinks, biscuits and processed foods, the fructose simply overloads the liver's glycogen stores and, because one of the by products of its metabolism stimulates the body to make fat, it is rapidly converted into fats called triglycerides. Some of these stay in the liver and build up as fatty deposits that damage the liver and ultimately adversely affect the way it works. Others find their way into the bloodstream, forming fatty deposits in our arteries and filling up fat cells. Strange as it may seem, even though it is a sugar, when we consume fructose we are in effect consuming fat. Around 30% of the fructose we eat ends up as fat. Over time weight and blood pressure increase and eventually metabolic syndrome kicks in.

Experiments consistently show that the consumption of fructose directly increases the amount of uric acid the body produces. Uric acid levels can increase between 1 - 3 ml/dl within a very short time of consuming it. Although the precise mechanism is not fully understood, what is known is that, unlike other sugars, fructose needs something called Adenosine Triphosphate (ATP) for its metabolism. Adenosine Triphosphate is found in all of our cells as it provides them with a source of energy. Fructose induces hyperuricemia through a complex process that causes cells to burn up their Adenosine Triphosphate very rapidly. It happens throughout the body, but it is particularly pronounced in the liver where most of the fructose is metabolised. The liver becomes depleted of energy and this causes inflammation and scaring of the liver. After consuming large amounts of fructose cells become starved of their energy and go into a state of 'shock'. Cell death can then follow, sometimes on a very large scale. The DNA and RNA inside the cells provides an immediate source of purines that can be readily converted into uric acid. When this happens the amount of uric acid in the immediate vicinity of the dead and damaged cells can be up to 100 times greater than the amount in our blood and this acts as a pro-inflammatory hormone that stimulates our immune system and sets it on 'high alert'.

At the present time fructose, particularly in the form of High Fructose Corn Syrup, HFCS, is regarded as being 'the bad boy' especially when it comes to gout and hyperuricemia. Many believe that it is the main causative factor. But High Fructose Corn Syrup is not all that different to table sugar, HFCS is 55% fructose and 45% glucose, table sugar is 50% fructose and 50% glucose. The bottom line is that no sugar is good, especially when it is consumed in large amounts, and it becomes even more damaging when it is consumed with large amounts of the wrong type of fat. However important fructose and its over consumption is, there are many other factors in our modern lives that can lead to the development of hyperuricemia.

## Can Free Radicals and Inflammation Increase Levels of Uric Acid?

This is something that to me seems quite obvious as it follows on from what we know about uric acid and how it works as an antioxidant and immune system regulator in the body. However, I have not seen this idea put forward anywhere else. I find this a little surprising. The basic concept is that uric acid levels rise slowly over time, possibly over a period of years, for three reasons;

- First, they rise because the body's levels of dietary antioxidants and the raw materials or 'building blocks' it needs to make its own endogenous antioxidants are insufficient to cope with the amount of free radicals and other potentially damage causing substances that are 'floating around' and causing cell damage or cell death. If this is true, it is reasonable to assume that uric acid levels would fall when the amount of antioxidants available increases or when the number of free radicals is reduced and as a consequence the need for antioxidants is reduced.
- Second, we know that the amount of uric acid in the vicinity of dead

and dying cells is 100 times greater than the amount in the blood, so when free radicals and other damage causing substances overwhelm our body's antioxidant defences and cause large scale cell death, large amounts of uric acid are released directly into the blood stream as part of our body's normal immune response.

- Third, the on going health issues associated with hyperuricemia result in a chronic low grade inflammation. This kind of inflammation keeps the body in a constant 'attack and repair' response. Immune cells take charge and there are serious consequences to this unchecked on going inflammation. Neutrophils, one of the types of cells involved in our body's inflammatory response, attack what they perceive to be outside invaders or damage causing substances with the massive production of free radicals throughout the body. This is a perfectly normal and healthy response. However, when this goes on for a long time the body's general immune response ends up being compromised, leading to many long term side effects.

Where the free radicals and damage causing substances come from will be dealt with in the next chapter. But before we move on we need to consider other ways in which free radicals can increase levels of uric acid and in some of these cases the free radicals come from the body itself.

## It's All About Balance.

We know that uric acid is a powerful antioxidant. However, in certain circumstances the end products of the uric acid being the 'good guy' can be damaging. An example of this is when uric acid prevents the 'peroxidation' of lipids and fats.

Xanthine Oxidase and the breakdown of purines into uric acid is an major source of Superoxide free radicals. Under normal balanced conditions these Superoxides are rendered harmless by one of the body's own endogenous antioxidants Superoxide Dismutase. If conditions are not balanced and the body does not have enough Superoxide Dismutase or it has insufficient 'raw materials' to make adequate supplies of Superoxide Dismutase, the excess Superoxide becomes a damaging substance by reacting with nitric oxide to form peroxinitrite. Peroxinitite is not a free radical as such but it is a powerful inflammatory oxidant and nitrating agent that is capable of damaging a wide range of biological molecules, including DNA and the fats that make up our cell walls.

Uric acid is an extremely powerful 'scavenger' of peroxynitrite. The uric acid is able to directly inactivate the peroxynitrite but in the process of doing this it is oxidised by the peroxynitrites to form free radicals of uric acid. Under normal balanced conditions these uric acid free radicals are eliminated by the Vitamin C that is also present and their potential damaging effect is neutralised. However, if there is not enough Vitamin C available to work with the uric acid the damaging effect of the uric acid free radicals remains unchecked and they damage or kill cells and in the process give rise to a state of oxidative stress.

A complicated process that is something of a 'vicious circle'. With inadequate supplies of Superoxide Dismutase the more uric acid we make the more uric acid and Vitamin C we need. What this does serve to illustrate though it that the human body is all about balance. The right chemicals need to be in the right place, in the right amount and at the right time.

## Why do we not excrete enough uric acid?

Ninety per cent of the cases of hyperuricemia are thought to be caused by the under excretion of uric acid. So why does the body not excrete enough uric acid?

### Insulin Resistance and Diabetes

In the 1960s, a series of studies linked hyperuricemia to insulin resistance, poor glucose tolerance and diabetes. At the time the reason for this was not fully understood. However, we now know far more, and it is an interesting 'vicious circle' of events.

Insulin is a hormone that is released by the pancreas in order to regulate the amount of glucose or 'blood sugar' that is circulating in our blood. So as glucose levels rise more insulin needs to be released. High levels of insulin are known to increase the amount of uric acid that is reabsorbed after it has been filtered out by the kidneys. This directly reduces the amount that is excreted and as a result uric acid levels rise. High levels of uric acid reduce the amount of nitric oxide we produce.

Insulin needs nitric oxide to regulate the uptake of glucose, so it makes sense that the body's natural response to low levels of nitric oxide is to produce more insulin in order for it to be able to regulate blood glucose levels.

As insulin levels rise, more uric acid is reabsorbed and less uric acid excreted. As uric acid levels rise less nitric oxide is produced so in order to regulate blood sugar more insulin is produced. To compound an already bad situation something else happens. Although the mechanism is not fully understood, high levels of insulin are known to have an adverse impact on how the kidneys work. They work less efficiently and as a consequence they excrete less uric acid. Ultimately, as diabetes sets in, they become damaged. Diabetes is known to be the most common cause of kidney disease. So the more insulin resistant an individual is the higher the concentration of uric acid becomes. It is not surprising that people with hyperuricemia and gout often display the classic trappings of poor glucose tolerance, insulin resistance and type II diabetes.

## Fructose - It Scores Twice!

As well as directly increasing levels of uric acid, fructose also reduces the amount of uric acid that our bodies excrete. It does this in three ways:-

- Fructose competes with uric acid for access to transport proteins in the kidneys and this means that less uric acid is excreted. The effect of this is increased in people with a hereditary (genetic) predisposition towards hyperuricemia and gout.
- One of the end products of the metabolism of fructose is lactic acid and lactic acid directly inhibits the excretion of uric acid. Other substances, including alcohol (ethanol) also produce lactic acid when they are metabolised and they have the same direct impact on the excretion of uric acid.
- When fructose causes cells to rapidly burn up their Adenosine Triphosphate they become damaged and they die. Dead and dying cells create inflammation. As well as causing damage to the liver this inflammation can also make the kidneys work less efficiently.

## Your Digestive Tract.

We know that about two thirds of the uric acid turned over daily is excreted by the kidneys but nearly all of the rest is eliminated by bacteria in the digestive tract. In the absence of suitable bacteria, the excretion of the uric acid is reduced. Unfortunately people who consume a typical 'Western Diet' of too much sugar, meat, over refined carbohydrates and only a small amount of vegetables and fibre often have a spectrum of bacteria in their digestive tract that does not function efficiently, especially when it comes to excreting uric acid. Believe it or not fructose can have a very damaging effect on the bacteria in our digestive tract.

## High Levels of Lead

High levels of lead are known to significantly impair kidney function and reduce the amount of uric acid that is excreted. While today an excessive amount of lead in our bodies and 'lead poisoning' are extremely rare, from an historical perspective this is interesting. Both Seneca and the Roman physician Galen (A.D. 131-200) documented the occurrence of gout and its possible link to diet and a lifestyle of 'excess'. They were both well aware of the dangers of lead but they never made the link between lead and gout.

The Romans used lead extensively in their water supply systems, in fact the words plumbing and plumber come from the Roman word *plumbus* meaning lead. Cooking utensils and tableware were made from pewter, a tin alloy that also contained lead, and this meant that lead could leach into their food. Their wine makers also used lead and lead lined pots. They added 'sugar of lead' or lead acetate to their food and wine to sweeten it, and in the case of wine, also preserve it. So Seneca and Galen were correct. The prevalence of gout in Roman society was without doubt linked to diet and lifestyle but not in quite the way they thought.

## What about the "The Disease of Kings"?

Well in the Middle Ages pewter was also widely used by the wealthy for cooking utensils and tableware. The poor had to make do with wooden and iron utensils. The really rich may have eaten from gold or silver plates but pewter was widely used 'below stairs' in the preparation and cooking of food. The wealthy also used lead glazed pottery and in the 16th and 17th Century they drank from lead crystal glasses. As sugar was in very short supply, like the Romans they also used 'sugar of lead' to sweeten their food and wine. Add to this cosmetics that were used to give both men and women the white face that was so desirable and you had a recipe for disaster, with lead slowly building up over the years to dangerously high levels. Ironically the richer a person was the more lead they inadvertently consumed.

## Does Age Play a Part?

The simple answer is yes. We know that the incidence of gout and hence hyperuricemia increases with age and there are many reasons for this. Not least is that as we get older our bodies do not function quite as well as they used to; our kidneys aren't as efficient as they used to be at excreting waste products and our pancreas isn't as efficient as it used to be at regulating the production of insulin. In addition the natural turnover of cells in our bodies increases as we get older and as these cells die they increase the load of uric acid that the body has to handle. There are also age related changes to the connective tissue in our joints that are likely to encourage the formation of crystals.

With time we all age, some faster then others. In 1956 a 'free radical theory of ageing' was proposed and over the years this has gained wide acceptance. It is a fact that the body's production of free radicals and free radical damage increases with age. However, scientists have now identified something that they believe speeds up the ageing process. Advanced Glycation End products, also known as AGE's or Glycotoxins, are relatively new players on the health and nutrition scene but they are now considered to be one of the primary factors in ageing and degenerative diseases. Not only do they damage cells and encourage inflammation and oxidative stress, they are also strongly associated with degenerative diseases like diabetes and reduced kidney function, all of which impair the way in which the kidneys work and excrete uric acid.

In terms of the enzyme Xanthine Oxidase which is needed to make uric acid, something also happens. We know that gout is more common in men than women and one of the reasons for this is the male sex hormone testosterone. As we get older we tend to accumulate iron, so the amount of iron in the body increases with age, especially in men, as the amount of iron in women of childbearing age is regulated by their menstrual cycle. Readily available iron activates Xanthine Oxidase and another metal in our bodies, copper, deactivates it, so copper effectively puts a sort of 'brake' on Xanthine Oxidase. Testosterone increases the half life of copper so for most men while they are young, things are in balance. However, as men age and the AGE's mentioned earlier can accelerate the ageing process, their levels of testosterone fall and as a consequence the amount of copper diminishes, the 'brake' is reduced and Xanthine Oxidase becomes more active, resulting in the potential for the body to make higher levels of uric acid.

Reduced levels of copper also have another effect that can make the increased production of uric acid even worse. When uric acid is produced superoxide free radicals are generated. Under normal balanced conditions these are neutralised by the body's antioxidant enzyme Superoxide Dismutase. However the body needs copper in order to make Superoxide Dismutase, it is a copper based antioxidant, so a reduction in the amount of available copper means a reduction in the amount of Superoxide Dismutase available and as a consequence more and more free radicals are produced.

## Does Lifestyle Play a Part in Hyperuricemia?

In a word yes, and the impact of lifestyle can be greater than you think.

### Our state of Mind:

Believe it or not stress can be a killer. Our body is hard wired to protect us from the threat of danger. It has a natural alarm system of 'fight or flight' so when we are angry, anxious, tense and generally on edge our bodies produce a surge of hormones that prepare us for the fight that lies ahead. They increase our heart rate, increase our blood pressure and give rise to a sudden boost of energy. Cortisol, the primary stress hormone, increases the amount of glucose in the blood stream and enhances the way our brain and body uses this glucose. In anticipation of any damage that is likely to occur it also alters our immune system and puts our body's inflammatory response onto high alert. The poor sleep quality and short sleep duration that comes with stress also lead to increased levels of inflammatory markers.

Simply having gout makes you feel stressed, not least because of the pain, the constant 'why me?' the fear of the next attack and the utter hopelessness of the situation you find yourself in. Breaking the stress cycle is no easy task.

The body's stress response system is usually self regulating but when stress in life is always present our body is over exposed to Cortisol and other stress hormones and these then begin to disrupt many of our body's processes, creating a state of chronic inflammation that weakens our immune system and interferes with proper glucose metabolism and the release of insulin. Ultimately this leads to insulin resistance and a general state of oxidative stress, all of which has the effect of increasing levels of uric acid.

### Smoking:

Apart from creating vast amounts of free radicals that put an immense load on your body's antioxidant defences, when you smoke you are also depleting your body of many of the essential vitamins and minerals it needs to make these antioxidant defences. All of this damages cells and contributes to increased oxidative stress and as a consequence the need for more uric acid.

### Being Over weight:

When it comes to hyperuricemia weight is a big factor. A Body Mass Index, BMI, above normal is one of the most important risk factors for hyperuricemia. In addition, there is a direct correlation between a high BMI and high levels of uric acid. Whether increased weight is a 'lifestyle' issue that is linked to lack of exercise or simply consuming more calories than your body needs is not clear. One thing is certain, if you are overweight you are probably close to becoming insulin resistant and even moderate amounts of carbohydrates can trigger a dangerous cascade of events that ultimately leads to metabolic syndrome and more uric acid.

### Dieting:

If you do decide to try to lose weight avoid starving yourself or using any of the starvation zero carbohydrate diets that are widely promoted. Why? These types of diet will impair the ability of your kidneys to excrete uric acid as they make your body produce ketones and these compete with uric acid for one of the transport proteins in your kidneys. So when it comes to gout and hyperuricemia a 'Feast and Fast' life style or a high protein zero carbohydrate diet should most definitely not be on the agenda.

### Dehydration:

Obvious as it may sound, dehydration and simply just not drinking enough water can be a another reason why we do not excrete enough uric acid.

### Exercise:

Or to be more precise the lack of it! How much exercise do you get each day? For the vast majority of us the answer is, 'not a lot'. Lack of exercise increases insulin sensitivity and it has a negative effect on our state of mind. It also increases inflammatory markers and weight gain, none of which are a good idea when you have hyperuricemia and gout.

## Do Genetics Play a Part in Hyperuricemia?

The simple answer is yes. For years we have known that hyperuricemia and gout 'runs in families' and we now know that certain ethnic groups are more likely to develop hyperuricemia and gout than others. The genes URAT1 and SLC2A9 are known to be major determinants of uric acid levels as they encode a protein that helps to transport uric acid in the kidneys. No doubt as we learn more about the human genome more will be identified.

However, people who are genetically predisposed to hyperuricemia and gout do not necessarily go on to develop it as there can be important interactions between genetic factors and lifestyle. The Maori of New Zealand are a clear example of this, and strangely, it was the story of the Maori that set me off on the trail of finding out whether there really was a link between diet, lifestyle and gout.

The Maori of New Zealand have a marked predisposition to develop hyperuricemia and gout because of a genetic peculiarity, a peculiarity that is in fact common to all of the indigenous South Pacific Islanders that are descended from the Taiwanese Aboriginals. However, there is no mention of gout among the Maori's before the 20th Century, in fact the first observations of gout were in the 1940's.

On Captain Cooke's first voyage to New Zealand he was accompanied by Joseph Banks, a scientist who is best known for his interest in botany and biology. However, Banks was also a medical doctor. Even though Vitamins were not discovered until 1912, in 1747 a Scottish naval surgeon named James Lind had made the observation that something in citrus fruit prevented scurvy. Cooke's expedition to Australia and New Zealand was the first time lime juice, rationed out on a daily basis, was used therapeutically on a voyage to prevent scurvy. One of Banks' jobs was to observe and record the general health of the crew.

Banks kept extensive diaries and he described the Maori as 'lean and strong' and showing no signs of disease or ill health. He even described their diet. These ancient Maori ate a diet of sweet potato, taro, fern roots, wild fruit and vegetables, oil from a native flax plant, fish, birds and eggs. They had no alcohol, no wheat or grains, no mammalian meat and no dairy products. They cooked their food by either wrapping it in leaves and burying it in hot pits in the ground or by boiling it in wooden troughs in water that was heated by hot stones. The European settlers came in the 1850's bringing with them wheat, cattle, sheep and pigs but the Maori kept to their traditional food and way of life. It was only after they were urbanised and introduced to beer, different cooking methods and a diet that was high in read meat and carbohydrates and low in vegetables, fish and poultry that an epidemic of obesity and gout developed. The drastic changes in their diet and the adoption of the urbanised lifestyle of the developed countries has led them to now have the highest prevalence of gout in the world.

The history of the Maori demonstrates that genetically predisposed people are more likely to develop hyperuricemia and as a consequence gout if they are exposed to changes in lifestyle and to what can best be described as a 'Western Diet'. This is further substantiated by Filipinos who, like the Maori's, are genetically predisposed to gout. They have a much higher incidence of gout when living in the USA than they do when living in their own country. The country with the fastest growing incidence of gout is Taiwan where the hitherto remote Taiwanese Aboriginals, the people from whom all of the South Sea Islanders are descended, are now becoming urbanised and as a consequence exposed to a 'Western Diet'.

So what, if any, are the links between diet, hyperuricemia and gout?

CHAPTER 8

# Are We Really What We Eat?

## Is There a Link Between Diet and Gout?

The interaction between food, body chemistry and our health is extremely complicated. There are many variables that can come into play. Genetics in particular can have a major impact on how our bodies metabolise the food we eat and how susceptible we are to disease. Did you know that there are about 100 genes known to be involved in the metabolism of cholesterol and that a variant of just one of these, CETP, can protect an individual against cardiovascular disease?

Much of what we do know about the relationship between diet and health is either the result of epidemiological studies undertaken over a period of years or laboratory experiments that try hard to mimic the human body. Most research into gout and the causes of gout is undertaken using genetically modified animals or 'In vitro' in Petri dishes, in a laboratory and under super controlled conditions. Despite everyone's best efforts the results from this type of 'in vitro' research can often not be replicated when they are undertaken 'in vivo' using people or animals in natural conditions. A rather simplistic illustration of this is the amount of Vitamin C in an apple. The average apple contains about 5mg of Vitamin C, yet the antioxidant effect of the apple when it is eaten is equivalent to that of a 1,500mg supplement of Vitamin C. Clearly there are other substances either in the apple or in our bodies that are in some way reinforcing the effect of the Vitamin C. In reality, despite an astoundingly rapid increase in our understanding of the human body and the human genome, we still have an lot to learn about the complex inter relationships between our health and the food we eat.

When it comes to understanding and writing about diet, nutrition and health many of us have a sort of unintentional 'hidden agenda'. As a consequence all too often we succumb to a sort of 'tunnel vision' and only see what we want to see. So the first thing we need to do is look at the facts and look at the evidence. What, if anything, do we actually know about the effect of diet on hyperuricemia and gout and if diet really does play a part, why is it having an effect now and why is this effect increasing at such an alarming rate.

If humans and the higher primates are the only mammals in which the end product of the metabolism of purines is uric acid, the first question we need to answer is "Do the higher primates suffer from gout"? The simple answer is no. Outside of the laboratory only humans spontaneously develop gout. This leads us to ask the second question, "Why do the higher primates not suffer from gout?"

If you compare uric acid levels in the higher primates to those of humans the figures are quite interesting; 1.5–3.0 mg/dl for the higher primates versus 6.0–6.5 mg/dl for humans. This current 'average' figure is for a healthy human who does not suffer from hyperuricemia. We know that uric acid levels in humans have risen significantly over the last half of the 20th Century but in the 1920s, the average uric acid level for Americans was about 3.5 mg/dl, a level that is fairly close to that of the higher primates. Now this leads us to ask the question, what has changed over the last 90 years? Certainly it is reasonable to assume that the moderate difference in levels of uric acid between the higher primates and the average American of the 1920's can be attributed to diet and lifestyle, but why has this difference increased so much in the later part of the 20th Century and why is it continuing to increase at such an alarming rate?

The diet of a higher primate consists mainly of raw vegetation and fruit. Occasionally they eat meat but overall their diet contains only small amounts of animal protein. Fruit and vegetables are eaten raw and the primates live an active life protected from free radicals and the sun's rays by their fur and dark skin, in an environment in which there is little or no air pollution and as a consequence few free radicals in the air they breathe. We know that fruit and vegetables in their natural state are mildly alkalising and anti inflammatory, so the body of the higher primate is 'in balance' and despite the absence of uricase and the existence of uric acid they live a gout free life.

So what evidence, if any, do we have that links our diet and the food we eat to hyperuricemia and gout? We know that iron is needed and that the consumption of large amounts of fructose has a definite effect on levels of uric acid, but are high levels of insulin, inadequate amounts of antioxidants and the presence of free radicals and other damage causing substances also linked to diet? If they are, how have our dietary habits changed over the last 80 to 90 years to bring about such a significant increase in the levels of uric acid found in the population of the Western world.

## Insulin: Why Are Insulin Levels Rising?

Our bodies produce insulin when we consume and metabolise carbohydrates. But what exactly are carbohydrates? Most of us immediately think of pasta, rice, bread and potatoes but carbohydrates come in many disguises. They are one of the most abundant biological molecules and they fulfil many roles. The food we eat supplies us with carbohydrates in two different forms, starch and sugar. Both of these contain fibre and cellulose. Starches and sugars provide us with energy. Fibre and cellulose provides us with the 'bulk' our digestive systems need to work efficiently. With the exception of the sugar fructose all carbohydrates, irrespective of whether they are starch or sugar, are digested and metabolised to into glucose and this is used throughout our body as a source of energy.

The amount of insulin circulating in our bodies is directly related to both the amount of carbohydrates we consume and the 'form' in which they are consumed. When they are complex they take longer to digest and metabolise. The more carbohydrates we consume the more insulin we need to keep glucose levels properly regulated. Over time cells become resistant to insulin so the pancreas needs to produce more in order to keep thing in check. In the end it is not able to produce enough insulin to control the amount of glucose in the blood. Eventually Metabolic Syndrome develops and then type II diabetes. If the pancreas becomes totally exhausted and loses it ability to produce insulin type I insulin dependent diabetes can result. It is not uncommon for adults to be somewhere between these two extremes, producing more insulin than normal but still able to keep their blood glucose within limits.

High levels of insulin correlate to glucose intolerance, insulin resistance and diabetes. Between one in three and one in four people in the west is now thought to be suffering from one of these conditions. Persistently high levels of insulin also block the breakdown of fat and this leads to weight gain and above normal body weight. This is close to becoming an epidemic even amongst children.

Carbohydrates are natural foods. They become unnatural when they are in a form, concentration or quantity that is not found in nature. In nature sweet and starchy things like fruit and carbohydrates are rare and they are usually only available for a short time of the year. The reason a lot of us crave sugar and carbohydrates is that from an evolutionary perspective they are quite rare nutrients and it was a good idea to eat a lot of them when you could. For early man fruit and tubers containing carbohydrate were usually only around in the autumn so we are wired to eat a lot, store them as fat and use the fat to help us to survive the winter when food was scarce.

Natural unrefined unprocessed carbohydrates come with loads of fibre, vitamins, minerals, water, antioxidants and phytonutrients. The water fills you up and the fibre slows the rate at which the carbohydrates are absorbed in the digestive tract and converted to glucose. This means that they create less of a 'sugar spike' in the blood and this has a direct impact on the amount and rate at which insulin is produced. The vitamins, antioxidants and phytonutrients are valuable as they are essential for our bodies to function properly and they also help prevent and repair cell damage.

## Starchy Carbohydrates:

Our ancestors, the early hunter gatherers, are thought to have consumed between 80 and 100 grams of starchy carbohydrates a day and these carbohydrate would have been in a complex unrefined form. It is estimated that the typical Western diet contains between 350-600 grams of carbohydrate a day, an increase of between 500% and 750%. Somehow our bodies have to cope with this massive increase.

However, in addition to the amount of carbohydrate that we consume, the type of carbohydrate has also changed. Instead of complex 'whole' carbohydrates that contain large amounts of fibre and micro nutrients we are now consuming highly refined carbohydrates and this has as much effect on insulin levels as the amount of carbohydrate itself. The slower the rate at which carbohydrates are absorbed and converted to glucose the less insulin the body needs to produce to regulate blood glucose levels.

Where do these refined carbohydrates come from in our diet? Bread, cakes, biscuits/cookies, breakfast cereals, crisps, chips/fries, rice, pasta; the list is endless and the carbohydrates are invariably 'empty', over refined and very low in nutritional value.

## The Carbohydrate Sugar:

Man's love affair with sugar goes back a long way and it plays an insidious role in our health. For some reason we are in a way 'wired' to seek it out. But if sugar is bad for us why do we crave it? The short answer is that like other 'tasty foods' sugar stimulates the same centres in our brain that respond to heroin and cocaine and just like these drugs it has a very pronounced effect. In reality sugar acts on our brain almost like an addictive drug.

Why this happens is interesting as it comes from a time in our evolutionary past when as a result of climate change sugar, in the form of fruit, was only available for a short time of the year. Millions of years ago our early ancestors lived in a tropical climate and were able to eat fruit containing sugar throughout the year. As they moved into Eurasia and the climate cooled the forests became deciduous and fruit was only available for a short time of the year. This resulted in hungry near starving apes and a species that was in decline. At some point a mutation occurred and this made some of the apes extremely efficient at processing the fructose that was found in the seasonal fruit. Even small amounts could be metabolised and very quickly stored as fat. This gave these apes a huge survival advantage. They ate a lot of fruit while they could, put on fat and used the fat to help them survive when food was scarce. Today all apes, including humans, have this mutation. Our bodies have evolved to survive on very little sugar. So when sugar, especially in its refined form, is available we get fat because we are in some way 'wired' to seek it out and we eat far too much of it.

In reality sugar is one of the first 'manufactured' foods. It was first domesticated on the island of New Guinea about 10,000 years ago. The raw sugar cane was chewed and it is thought that the juice extracted from the cane was used in religious ceremonies. Sugar spread slowly from island to island reaching mainland Asia around 1,000BC. By 500AD it had reached India where it was used as a medicine. By 600AD it had spread to Persia and when the Arab armies conquered Persia they took a love of sugar and the knowledge of how to make it back to the Middle East. As the Arab Empire grew, wherever they went sugar went with them and they more or less turned sugar refining into an industry.

Probably the first Europeans to come across sugar were the Crusaders and the first sugar began reaching Europe in small amounts. It was regarded as a spice. It was expensive and only consumed by the wealthy. Some enterprising Crusaders saw an opportunity and began farming and processing sugar cane in small quantities in Cyprus but as the Crusades ended the supplies from the Arabs diminished new sources of supply were needed. The hunt was on to find places where sugar cane could be grown and it soon found its way via the Canary and Cape Verde Islands to the Caribbean. As more sugar cane was planted and refined the price of sugar fell and as the price fell so consumption and demand increased. The rest, as they say, is history.

In 1700 the average Englishman consumed 4 pounds of sugar a year. By 1800 he was eating 18 pounds a year and by 1870 consumption had risen to 47 pounds. By 1900 we were consuming 100 pounds a year. Today, about 25 percent of people on a typical 'Western Diet' consume around 95 kilograms or getting on for 200 pounds of sugar a year and for most of us this is more than our body weight. Sounds impossible? Well not when you consider that a 12 ounce can of 'regular' soft drink can contain up to 10 teaspoons of sugar, a massive 40 grams which is just under one and a half ounces.

## So what exactly is sugar?

First and foremost sugar is a natural food. It only becomes unnatural when it is in a form, concentration or quality that is not found in nature. Sugar comes in several forms and many disguises. The most common form is sucrose or what we know as table sugar. This is a 'dissacharide', a compound that is made up of one molecule of glucose that is linked to one molecule of fructose. So it contains 50% glucose and 50% fructose. When it is metabolised it is converted into separate molecules of glucose and fructose. These are both simple sugars or 'monosaccharides'. There is a third monosaccharide galactose. All other types of sugar are made from these three monosaccharides.

## A voice in the wilderness

In the 1960's a British nutrition expert called John Yudkin conducted a series of experiments on animals and people that showed that high amounts of sugar in their diet led to high levels of fat and insulin in the blood, risk factors he believed to be for heart disease and diabetes. But Yudkin's message was drowned out by the chorus of other scientists who were blaming the rising rates of obesity, heart disease and diabetes on the high levels of cholesterol that resulted from the consumption of too much saturated fat. As a consequence we were told to reduce the amount of saturated fat we were eating and as a result, saturated fat now makes up a smaller proportion of the average American diet than it did 40 years ago. So what filled the gap in fat consumption? Unsaturated fats in the form of vegetable oils and margarine, but despite this the number of people who are overweight or obese has not reduced. In reality it has grown larger and the incidence of heart disease and diabetes has increased at an alarming rate.

## Where does sugar come from in our diet?

Sugary soft drinks, biscuits, cakes, cookies, confectionery and surprisingly processed and manufactured foods. Why processed and manufactured foods? Sugar is a wonderful preservative so it is used in large quantities as a preservative. It is also used as a 'browning' agent, on the basis that colour equals flavour. In the west we have become addicted to 'brown', 'caramelised' food.

So what about the Maori? Well they had no sugar other than that occurring naturally in their fruit and vegetables and these were all seasonal. Their carbohydrates were complex and unrefined and they came from the sweet potatoes and taro that they had brought with them a thousand years earlier when they migrated from other South Pacific islands. They also ate the roots of native ferns and interestingly, highly nutritious varieties of purple and orange potatoes that were given to them by Captain Cooke.

## Fructose and High Fructose Corn Syrup.

Fructose, also called fruit sugar, occurs naturally both on its own as a monosaccharide and also as one of the molecules that table sugar, (sucrose), is made from. High Fructose Corn Syrup (HFCS) is a manufactured product that is 55% fructose and 45% glucose. Fructose is the only carbohydrate known to directly increase levels of uric acid and because of this, for many who write about diet and gout, it has become something of a "bête noire", especially when it is in the form of High Fructose Corn Syrup.

Fructose is a simple sugar that is found in varying amounts in fruit and vegetables, either on its own as a monosaccharide or combined with glucose as a disaccharide. When vegetables and fruit are eaten as a 'whole food' and in normal amounts the nutrients, antioxidants, fibre and other compounds that they contain counter any detrimental effect of the fructose as the fibre means that it is absorbed slowly into our bodies. So a small amount of fructose is not a bad thing. In fact, there is some evidence that a little bit may help your body process glucose properly. However, consuming too much fructose, especially when it is in a pure refined form appears to overwhelm the body's ability to process it.

The fructose in HFCS is no different to the fructose found in other foods. Once inside your body fructose works in the same way irrespective of whether it comes from corn syrup, cane sugar, strawberries, onions, or tomatoes. Only the amounts of fructose are different. For example, a cup of chopped tomatoes has 2.5 grams of fructose, a medium size desert apple about 4.5 grams, a 300ml can of non-diet soft drink contains around 23 grams, and a 'super-size' soft drink has about 62 grams. From a health perspective it is strongly recommended that your daily consumption of fructose is less than 25 grams, in other words the amount found in five desert apples or one 300ml can of non diet or 'regular' soft drink. The diets of our ancestors contained only very small amounts of fructose and it was only consumed for short periods of the year when fruit and berries were ripe. They used it to build up their fat reserves for the winter. Today it is estimated that about 10% of the calories in a modern 'Western' diet comes from fructose. Of the 152 pounds of 'sugar' the average American consumes each year 64 pounds is thought to be fructose in the form of High Fructose Corn Syrup.

When it comes to fructose and sugar we are being well and truly 'conned' into thinking that certain foods are healthy when they are not. Honey is presented as a healthy option, presumably because it is 'natural' and contains some beneficial nutrients, but it has about the same fructose to glucose ratio as high fructose corn syrup. Fruit juice is widely promoted as being one of your "5 a day" and a healthy way to start your day. Not true. Notwithstanding that the processing of these juices strips away most of their nutritional value, they contain a lot of fructose and no fibre. A 100 gram portion of a whole orange contains 1.5grams of fibre and 6.4 grams of sugar, of this sugar 1.9 grams is fructose. A 100 gram portion of orange juice however contains no fibre and 10 grams sugar, of this sugar 3 grams is fructose. Doesn't sound too bad? Well it does when you consider that the average orange weighs about 150 grams and the average glass of fruit juice is 300ml i.e. 300g. The whole orange provides 2.2 grams of fibre and 9.6 grams of sugar of which 1.9 grams is fructose while the orange juice provides no fibre and 30 grams of sugar and 9 grams of this is fructose. In other words 3 times as much sugar and around 4 times as much fructose. Fruit juice concentrates are also widely used as 'healthy' sweeteners. Look at the ingredients on the labels of packaged foods and you will invariably see sugar in one form or another. In reality finding manufactured food that does not contain sugar is actually quite difficult. As food manufacturers use the generic term sugar most people have no idea which products fructose is in or how much of it they are consuming.

Why our consumption of fructose has increased at such an alarming rate over the last thirty to forty years is the subject of a considerable amount of speculation. It is easy to become a little cynical about it. In America, because of corn subsidies, High Fructose Corn Syrup became incredibly cheap, much cheaper than conventional sugar. As it is fairly concentrated and in a liquid form that is easy to transport, it quickly found its way into a vast number of the foods we eat every day. Its introduction into the Western diet in 1975 was a multi-billion dollar boon for the corn industry. Almost all manufactured and packaged, processed foods now have sugar added in some form or other and this almost always includes fructose. Just to get some idea of the scale, 240,000 tonnes of fructose are produced each year. A massive amount. Not only is it added to food and drinks, it is also used in large quantities as a 'browning' agent in many manufactured and processed foods and this, in particular, is of great concern as people are unaware that they are consuming sugar. Another issue that needs to be kept in mind is that High Fructose Corn Syrup is almost invariably made from genetically modified corn. Some people have expressed concerns about genetically modified or "GM" foods. While the jury is still out on GM foods it could mean that HFCS brings with it another new set of as yet unknown dangers.

Over the past few years HFCS has been gathering something of a 'bad press' and as a consequence the consumption of both HFCS and sugar is falling slowly. So where do we go from here? Well the corn industry has come up with another product, "crystalline fructose" that is being used in soft drinks. This is produced by allowing fructose to crystallize out from a fructose-enriched corn syrup. This produces a product that is 99.5 percent pure fructose. In other words it contains nearly twice as much fructose as the HFCS currently being used. To make matters worse it is being promoted as being in some way 'healthier', a "pure fruit sugar" that is and better for you than HFCS. Clearly, all the health problems associated with HFCS could become even more pronounced when this product becomes widely used.

There is no doubt that in the Western World we are consuming vast amounts of fructose. Where does fructose come from in our diet? As with all sugars it is present in very large amounts in manufactured foods. In fact it is in almost all of the food that we consume that is not in a 'natural' form. And it shows up is some surprising places, even things that are not 'sweet' like sliced bread and processed meats contain it. Next time you buy a tin of chopped tomatoes check the label. You may be surprised!

## What About Antioxidants?

Our bodies need antioxidants and they make every effort to stay saturated with them. The antioxidants in our bodies come from two sources:-

- Antioxidants that our bodies make, the "Endogenous" antioxidants; catalase, superoxide dismutase, glutathione peroxidase, alpha lipoic acid, Coenzyme Q10, melatonin, ferritin, bilirubin are just some of them and of course there is also uric acid.
- Antioxidants that we obtain directly from the food we eat, "Exogenous" antioxidants like Vitamin C and Vitamin E along with Vitamin A which our body makes from the beta carotenes.

All foods, including meat, poultry, fish and eggs contain antioxidants, but the amount of antioxidant contained in each food varies tremendously. Not all antioxidants are created equal either and they do not work in the same way. Some are expert at fighting certain types of free radicals, some like uric acid and Vitamin C are water soluble and work in our blood and some like Vitamin E are fat soluble and work inside our cells. Some like Alpha lipoic acid work as a 'regulator' that restores the antioxidant properties of Vitamin C and Vitamin E after they have neutralised free radicals in our bodies.

Most of us are familiar with antioxidants like Vitamin C and Vitamin E but in total there are around 8,000 different antioxidants; beta carotene, the precursor of Vitamin A, is an antioxidant and minerals and trace elements like selenium, zinc, copper, manganese and the amino acids methionine and cysteine all play a part in helping our bodies remove unwanted free radicals. Lycopine, Zeaxanthin, Resveratrol, flavonoids such as quercetin and the anthocyanins, all form part of our body's antioxidant army. The list is enormous. The entire plant kingdom is teeming with antioxidants; beans, nuts, seeds and grains as well as vegetables and fruit all contain large quantities and they provide both the raw materials or 'building blocks' that our body needs to make its own antioxidants and the source of the antioxidants we need to obtain directly from our food.

How strong are the antioxidants in various foods? A difficult question to answer. The total amount of antioxidant found in a fruit or vegetable used to be measured by its ORAC score as this was thought to be the best measure of antioxidant capacity. The higher the ORAC score, the more antioxidant the fruit or vegetable contained. However the ORAC score is no longer regarded as being entirely accurate so other methods of assessing antioxidant values such as FRAP are being used. As a general rule the more brightly coloured a vegetable or piece of fruit is the better its health giving properties, so the advice to 'eat a rainbow' really does hold true. The precise amount of antioxidant in a specific food is to a some extent not really relevant. The more fruit and vegetables we eat, the more 'complete' they are and the less they are cooked, the more antioxidants and other essential micro nutrients and minerals our bodies are able to obtain from them. The current advice to eat at least '5 a day' has plenty of scientific evidence to support it.

One thing that we easily loose sight of is that we are very closely related to the higher primates and a primate's diet is almost exclusively vegetables and fruit, animal protein is a long way down the list. In terms of our digestive tract we are much closer to a herbivore than a carnivore. Meat eating animals have a digestive tract that is about three times the length of their body and this ensures that food does not stay in their body for long. Because it takes a long time for the nutritional content of vegetables to be absorbed, the digestive tract of a herbivore is ten to twelve times its body length. Our digestive tract is just like the herbivores, twelve times our body length. Our body needs protein and this protein can come from meat, fish, poultry, eggs or vegetables. There is nothing wrong with the protein coming from animal sources provided it comes in moderate quantities. Vegetables and fruit however are essential and we need them in large quantities if our bodies are to work properly and our digestive tract work efficiently.

In the Western world and in America in particular, the dietary intake of vegetables and fruit is at an all time low. According to the UCLA Centre for Human Nutrition, the four most commonly consumed fruit and vegetable in America are: 1 - French fries, 2 - Ketchup, 3 - Pizza sauce and 4 - Iceberg lettuce. Only about 5% of the population eat 5 daily servings of fruit and vegetables. The average consumption of fruit and vegetables is only 1.4 servings a day. Only 17% of the population eat 2 to 4 servings a day and only 12% of the population have what could be called a "good" or healthy diet.

The reasons for this? Well frequency of shopping may have something to do with it as you need to shop more frequently if you are to maintain an adequate supply of fruit and vegetables. Many of us are also intrinsically lazy and vegetables take time to prepare and cook. Historically meat was expensive so vegetables were eaten almost by default as they were all people could afford. As farming became 'industrialised' and animals were intensively reared and fed on grain as opposed to grass, the cost of meat reduced and this resulted in more meat being eaten. In reality some of us just simply don't like the taste or texture of fruit and vegetables. A more likely reason though is that many of us have acquired a taste for and are now addicted to fast food and junk food, both of which satisfy the craving for carbohydrates that so many of us seem to be wired with.

How much 'antioxidant' do we need in order to keep ourselves healthy and gout free? Its impossible to say. Antioxidants are needed to combat the adverse effects of free radicals and the amount of free radicals we are exposed to depends not only on the food we eat and how the food is cooked, but also the environment in which we live, the quality of the air we breath, the amount of sunlight we are exposed to and the general state of our health.

What about the Maori? Well before they were urbanised they consumed plenty of antioxidants in the form of vegetables, that were either eaten raw or steamed or boiled. Once they became urbanised however, their consumption of vegetables reduced significantly and combined with other diet and lifestyle changes the end result was gout.

## Too Much Iron: 'Iron Overload'

Iron is needed to make Xanthine Oxidase and high levels of iron can stimulate the production of uric acid. In addition, we know that in the absence of uric acid iron 'binds' to Vitamin C and makes it inactive. This has the effect of reducing the amount of Vitamin C that is available. Do high levels of iron have other consequences in terms of our health?

Iron is an essential nutrient and for years a lack of it caused one of the most common nutritional deficiencies, anaemia. However, in the Western world more attention is being paid these days to the opposite problem, iron overload, which some people have linked to an increased risk of diabetes, coronary heart disease and cancer. In a recent study of 1,000 white Americans between the age of 67 and 96, 13% had levels of iron that were considered high and only 3% were considered to be deficient in iron. In the western world iron deficiency in men and post menopausal women is rare.

Our body handles iron very carefully, to the extent that it even recycles it from old red blood cells. Recycling is essential as the human diet historically contained only just enough iron to replace the small amount that is lost each day. Our body is also able to regulate the 'uptake' of iron; the less iron you have the more iron your body absorbs, likewise the more iron you have the less it absorbs. Because iron is so important our body guards its store of iron very carefully, so carefully in fact that it has no way of excreting it. Each day we only need a trace amount of iron to replace the tiny amount that we lose. Even for an adult man this is as little as 1mg to 2mg a day. Because the body is unable to completely shut down the absorption process the more iron we consume and absorb from our food the higher the level of stored iron becomes. Short of a blood donation, the body just can’t get rid of it.

Even without a rare genetic disorder (Hemochromatosis ) that leads to the accumulation of very high levels of iron, stored iron can cause health problems. In a 10 years study of 32,000 women, those who consumed the most iron, and as a consequence had the highest levels of stored iron, were nearly three times more likely to have diabetes than those with the lowest levels of iron. In another study of 38,000 men, those who consumed the most iron had a 63% greater risk of developing diabetes. Now this begs the question of whether is it the actual iron or other things in the food containing the iron that was causing the diabetes. It could also be that other foods consumed with the iron rich food, a steak with chips/fries for instance, were contributing to the problem. However, other studies have since shown that when people with high levels of stored iron donate blood on a regular basis, their insulin sensitivity and risk of diabetes diminishes. Why? Put simply iron overload damages the pancreas and affects its ability to produce insulin, so the end result for some is insulin resistance and diabetes, both of which can cause an increase in levels of uric acid.

## Where Does The Iron In Our Diet Come From?

Meat, fish, poultry, eggs and vegetables all contain iron. However there are two different types of iron. HEME iron is a type of iron that is derived from red blood cells and it is only found in meat, fish and poultry. Non HEME iron is found in vegetables and fruit as well as animal products. HEME iron is much more easy to absorb than non HEME iron. Whereas between 15% and 30% of HEME iron is absorbed, only about 5% of non HEME iron finds its way into the blood. Interestingly, the uptake of the non HEME iron is much better regulated by the body than the uptake of the HEME iron, so the accumulation of iron and iron 'over load' is more likely if your diet is high in the iron found in animal products.

Various factors can influence the way in which iron is absorbed and not least of these is gender. Pre menopausal women absorb iron much more efficiently than men; from a similar meal they will absorb around three times as much as a man and when they are pregnant this figure can increase to around nine times. Vitamin C, some of the proteins found in meat, and acids naturally present in many fruits and vegetables can all increase the absorption of the non HEME iron found in vegetables, sometimes by as much as 85%. Alcohol and sugar consumption enhance the absorption of both types of iron. While Vitamin C has a neutral effect on how HEME iron is absorbed, some vegetables like spinach, that contain oxalic acid can interfere with and slow down the absorption of

HEME iron. High fibre whole grains that contain phytates and foods that are high in calcium also reduce the amount of iron that is absorbed. So it would appear that the more vegetables you eat the less HEME iron your body is able to take on board. Where else does the iron in our diet come from? Probably as a legacy from the past, when dietary iron was in short supply, most manufactured food is now enriched with iron; flour, breakfast cereals, breads, pasta, even infant formula and baby foods are all fortified with iron and many of us also take daily vitamin supplements without realising that they also contain iron.

Not so long ago, before farming became a semi industrialised process with huge animal feeding operations, the price of meat and poultry was high. Only the wealthy could afford to eat it every day. For most people meat was something of a luxury that was only consumed once or twice a week and even then, it was only consumed in modest amounts. However, with the advent of intensive farming methods the price of meat dropped and as a consequence consumption has soared. In 1961 the world's total meat supply was estimated to be 71 million tons. By 2007, it had risen to 284 million tons. When you allow for world population growth and real changes in global GDP, this represents a 70% increase. Per capita consumption has more than doubled over that period. In developing countries it has risen twice as fast, doubling in the last 20 years.

Americans are now consuming close to 276 pounds of meat, poultry and fish per person per year and getting on for half of this is red meat. Australians are consuming almost as much but in Luxembourg the figure is even higher; 300lbs or just over 140kg per person per year. Not surprisingly India has the lowest consumption of meat at 7 pounds, just over 3 kilos a person. 276 pounds of meat a year works out at just under 12 ounces or 350 grams of meat, poultry or fish a day. Red meat contains around 3.7mg iron per 100 grams, fish and poultry around 1.3mg. So if you consume 350 grams of animal protein a day that's just under 13mg from red meat and 4.5mg from poultry and fish. As getting on for half of our animal protein consumption is from red meat, that averages out at around 8.75mg of iron a day.

## How much iron do we need on a daily basis?

Well, we know that a healthy man only actually needs between 1mg and 2mg of iron a day, so to allow for the fact that only some of the iron we consume is absorbed the recommended daily guideline is 8mg a day for men and post menopausal women and 18mg a day for pre menopausal women. When you look at these figures 8.75mg a day from animal protein doesn't look too bad. However, other foods like bread, breakfast cereals, flour and pasta are all fortified with iron. Because so many nutrients are taken out in the milling and refining process, in most countries white bread is fortified with enough iron to bring it to within 80% of the amount of iron that is naturally found in whole grain bread, 3.6mg per 100 grams. Now because the fibre and phytates in whole grain bread reduce the absorption of iron, this amount of iron isn't too much of a problem, but in white bread there is very little fibre and no phytates. An average slice of white bread weighs around 70 grams, that's 2.5mg of iron. How much bread does the average person consume each day? A lot more than one slice. Breakfast cereal contains anything upwards of 10mg of iron per 100 grams. Even with the recommended serving of just 30 grams this means that 3.3mg of iron are added to the daily iron load and many of us actually eat portions of breakfast cereal that are nearer to 50 or 70 grams. If you include bread, pasta and other fortified foods it is easy to see how the recommended daily allowance for iron of 8mg a day is easily exceeded. Just one average portion of animal protein, 2 slices of white bread and 30 grams of breakfast cereal will deliver just over 19mg, more than twice the recommended daily amount. How much of this iron is actually absorbed is another matter, but it is clear that with such an abundant supply of iron slowly, over a number of years, it is easy for iron to accumulate to a level that will potentially cause health problems.

So with the widespread consumption of large quantities of animal proteins, iron enriched processed foods and a diet that is low in vegetables, fruit and fibre, many people in the Western world now have levels of stored iron that are higher than they should be. In addition to stimulating Xanthine Oxidase and the production of uric acid, this iron also increases the risk of developing insulin resistance and diabetes, both of which reduce the excretion of uric acid and contribute to the development of hyperuricemia.

Red meat, especially organ meats, contains high levels of purines and purines are the building blocks from which uric acid is made. As a consequence for centuries the consumption of red meat has been linked to gout. From an epidemiological perspective the link between meat, poultry and fish consumption and gout is inevitable as animal protein is a major component of a "Western diet". However, this diet is also high in sugar, over refined carbohydrates, processed foods and vegetable oils and it is extremely low in fresh fruit and vegetables. As a consequence despite everyone's best efforts it is almost impossible to separate the consumption of meat from the consumption of the other foods and prove any direct cause and effect relationships. However, when you look at iron and the sources of iron in our diet it is clear that there is an undeniable link between hyperuricemia and the consumption of animal protein. Somewhat ironically and contrary to conventional dietary advice, this is not because of the purines that these animal proteins contain, it is the iron. Purines appear to be innocent bye standers.

## What about the Maori?

Well, prior to the arrival of the European settlers and their urbanisation around 100 years ago, while they roamed their tribal lands their diet contained fish, poultry in the form of wild birds, eggs and fish eggs, lots of vegetables and some complex carbohydrates found in taro, sweet potatoes and fern roots. They had no mammalian meat. Their health problems began when they stopped eating fish, poultry, vegetables and complex carbohydrates and started drinking alcohol, eating refined carbohydrates and large amounts of red meat.

## Free Radicals & Other Damaging Substances

Where do the Free Radicals, Reactive Oxygen Species (ROS) and other damage causing substances come from? Free radicals and ROS are impossible to avoid. Each day our body is exposed to millions of them and they come from many different sources. Free radicals are formed when our bodies are exposed to the sun's rays and they are in the air we breath and in the water we drink. Air pollution, environmental chemicals, cigarette smoke, alcohol and stress all contribute to our daily free radical load. All of the food we eat contains free radicals and just as our body makes its own antioxidants, it also produces free radicals, many of which are essential in controlled amounts for life and health. Our immune cells use free radicals to destroy invading foreign organisms and there is also evidence that they play an important part in how our cells work. Free radicals are a by product of simply 'living'.

As with antioxidants, free radicals are not created equal. Some have the capacity to cause far more damage than others. The more free radicals we are exposed to the more antioxidants our bodies need to keep them in check. Under normal balanced conditions free radicals are rendered harmless either by our body's own antioxidants or by the antioxidants we consume in our food. However, if we are not consuming enough antioxidants or enough of the raw materials or building blocks that our bodies need to make its own antioxidants, the damaging effect of the free radicals remains unchecked. Our body's defences are overwhelmed and this leaves us vulnerable to cell damage, oxidative stress and disease. At the end of the day, the key to good health is about minimising the number of free radicals we are exposed to and ensuring that we have enough antioxidants to neutralise the ones we are exposed to.

Because it contains a lot of processed food, over refined carbohydrates, large amounts of animal protein and relatively small amounts of vegetables and fruit, a typical Western diet is high in free radicals and low in antioxidants. While some foods contain more free radicals than others and foods metabolise to produce free radicals in different ways, the way in which food is cooked can have just as much effect on the generation of free radicals as the food itself.

When it comes to the food that our Western diet contains we are living in an age of what can politely be called 'Misinformation'. Put less politely we are simply being 'conned' by a food manufacturing industry that is worth billions of dollars a year. We are told that things are good for us and that they are 'the healthy option' yet in reality they are not only not healthy, they are also actually bad for us. Fruit juice for breakfast is a classical example of this. It is not a healthy option and it most definitely does not count towards your '5 a day'. There are in fact a raft of foods that we consume every day that we should simply not be eating. Not only are they loaded with free radicals, they also adversely effect the way our body produces its own endogenous antioxidants and they have the potential to seriously damage our health; polyunsaturated vegetable oils, hydrogenated oils in the form of trans fats, over refined carbohydrates and processed meats are just some. The list is very long and the vast majority are foods that have crept stealthily into our diets over the last hundred years. Included below is information on what I think are the two most dangerous of the culprits: Polyunsaturated Vegetable Oils and Hydrogenated Vegetable Oils or Trans Fats.

## Polyunsaturated Vegetable Oils

If you asked the question which is worse for your health, white flour, sugar or polyunsaturated vegetable oils, most people would answer white flour or sugar. But are they really the bad guys they are made out to be? They have both been around for quite a while. Just look at some Victorian and Edwardian cookbooks. People ate them then and they were generally far healthier than we are today. In reality white flour and sugar are not fundamentally bad. What is bad is the enormous amounts of them that we are now consuming. Polyunsaturated vegetable oils on the other hand are something that did not exist a hundred years ago. They are entirely new and entirely unnatural foods and because of the damage they can cause, they are being described by some as the 'health villains' of the 20th Century.

## Why are Polyunsaturated Vegetable Oils bad for us?

Put simply our bodies are unable to handle them, especially in the amounts we are currently consuming them in. Our bodies need polyunsaturated vegetable oils but only in very small quantities. For almost all human history they have been consumed only in the small amounts that occur naturally in nuts and seeds, and nuts and seeds are complex foods that contain many other nutrients as well as the polyunsaturated vegetable oils. It is only since industrialised extraction processes came onto the scene that we have eaten them in large quantities. In order to understand why polyunsaturated vegetable oils are so bad we first need to understand what they are and where they fit into the big picture of fats and oils.

The technical or scientific name for fats and vegetable oils is 'fatty acids'. 'Lipids' is the medical name that is used to describe them. They are a class of organic substances that are not soluble in water. In simple terms they are made from chains of carbon and hydrogen atoms that are 'bound' together in different ways and held together at one end by a sort of ''head' that is made from carbon and oxygen atoms. The chains come in different lengths, they are twisted together and 'bent' in different ways and they come with different degrees of 'saturation'. A fat is 'saturated' when all of the available atoms of carbon and hydrogen are linked together and this makes them very stable. Because they are stable they do not oxidise or become 'rancid' even when they are heated for cooking purposes. As a general rule the more saturated a fat is the more stable it is and the more beneficial and safer it is to eat.

Fats and oils can be divided into three groups;

- Saturated fats:These have no free atoms of hydrogen, do not oxidise easily and are solid at room temperature.
- Monounsaturated fats: These have two hydrogen atoms missing and are usually liquid at room temperature. Like saturated fats they are relatively stable and do not oxidise or go rancid easily.
- Polyunsaturated fats: These have four or more hydrogen atoms missing and are liquid even when cold. These oils are very unstable and highly reactive. Even in their natural state they oxidise and go

rancid easily and this is why nature has packaged them up neatly inside nuts and seeds with their own supply of antioxidants and vitamins to protect them. As a consequence once they are extracted they become chemically highly reactive and are characterised by free radicals.

Polyunsaturated fats and oils are referred to as PUFA's. They are found in different amounts in all natural foods including meat, fish, vegetables and seeds. In general, vegetable oils such as sunflower, safflower, corn, soy, flax seed, sesame seed, pumpkin seed and canola or rapeseed oils are the most concentrated sources of PUFA's in our diet. These oils contain different types of fats in different proportions and they are broadly classified into 4 groups; Omega 3, Omega 6, Omega 9 and Conjugated fatty acids. Some, like Omega-3 and Omega-6, are essential for our body to work properly. As our body is unable to make these fats they are called "essential" fatty acids or EFA's and these need to be obtained from the food we eat.

## Essential Fatty Acids or EFA's:

Most of us have heard about essential fatty acids, the names Omega-3 and Omega-6 usually come to mind. But what exactly are they and why are they so important?

The Omega 3 and Omega 6 groups of fatty acids each contain a number of different fatty acids, most of which the body is either able to make or obtain directly from food. In order to make fatty acid in the Omega 3 group it needs the 'parent' Omega 3 fatty acid, Alpha Linolenic Acid (ALA). In order to make Omega 6 fatty acids it needs the 'parent' Linoleic Acid (LA).

- Omega 3: Alpha Linolenic Acid (ALA) is converted by the body into eicosapentaenoic acid (EPA) and decosahexaenoic acid (DHA). Unfortunately this conversion process is not very efficient and some scientists believe that as little as 1% of the Alpha Linolenic Acid we consume ends up as DHA and EPA. This 1% conversion rate decreases even more as we get older. Luckily both DHA and EPA can also be obtained directly from our food so we need to obtain a lot of DHA and EPA as well as ALA from our diet in order to make up for this poor conversion process. Unfortunately the modern Western diet does not provide a very good source of Omega 3 fats.

- Omega 6: Linoleic Acid (LA) is converted into Gamma-linolenic acid (GLA) and Arachidonic Acid (AA). Unlike ALA it is readily converted into GLA and AA and our Western diet provides an abundant source of Linoleic Acid.

In the early 1900's most of the fat in our diet was saturated or monounsaturated. It came mainly from butter, lard, beef fat, coconut or palm oil and in some parts of the world olive oil. Over the last three or four decades most of us have been led to believe that saturated fats are bad and that vegetable oils are good. Not true. Any dietary fat or oil can become harmful if it is oxidised and polyunsaturated oils are more likely to be damaged by being oxidised than anything else. Today most of the fat in our diet is polyunsaturated and in the form of soy, corn, sunflower, safflower and canola oil. The detrimental effect these fats have on our health is clear and well established, yet most of us still believe that they are the healthy option, as indeed I once did.

In all mammals cell tissues are made up mainly of saturated and monounsaturated fats. Omega 3 and Omega 6 fats are only needed in relatively small amounts. What makes polyunsaturated vegetable oils so bad for us is the large amount of them we now consume and as a consequence the residual amount that we have in our bodies. PUFA's are essentially unstable and easily affected by things around them. Too many PUFA's are increasingly incorporated into cell membranes and because they are unstable the cells then become fragile and prone to oxidation. This leads to cell damage, the generation of free radicals, inflammation and more uric acid.

## Saturated Fats:

Under normal conditions the saturated fats found in butter, eggs, cheese and meat are not easily oxidised. The cholesterol and essential fatty acids these foods contain are nutrients that provide the raw materials our bodies need to make a large number of hormones and enzymes as well as vitamin D. They also play a major part in helping to build our body's antioxidant defence team. Notwithstanding that many of us have been led to believe that cholesterol and saturated fats are 'bad', in reality our bodies are desperately in need of them. They are needed to build brain and nerve tissue, they nourish the immune system, they help regulate our mood and they are one of the building blocks for oestrogen and testosterone.

With the exception of a few people who have a gene that predisposes them to develop high levels of 'bad' HDL cholesterol, for most of us it is perfectly safe to consume reasonable amounts of saturated fats, provided they are part of a 'healthy' diet and are consumed with plenty of vegetables and fruit.

Contrary to what we have been told, saturated fats are not the "bad guys". Our bodies really do need them. They are an essential part of living and when they are replaced by other less healthy fats things can start going wrong. One of the interesting things about them is that to a certain extent our brain in a way 'runs' on them, so when they are in short supply it steals them from other parts of our body in order to keep going. Two things that suffer are oestrogen and testosterone, and we know from previous chapters that low levels of these hormones can have a direct impact on the amount of uric acid our body produces.

## Monounsaturated Fats:

The monounsaturated fatty acid most commonly found in our food is oleic acid which is the main component of olive oil. It is also found in the oils from almonds, pecans, cashews, peanuts and avocados. Olive oil contains 75% oleic acid, 13% saturated fat in the form of Palmitic acid, 10% omega-6 and 2% omega-3. It is also rich in polyphenols which have antioxidant, anti-inflammatory, anti-clotting and anti-bacterial properties. It is an oil that has withstood the test of time and it is the safest vegetable oil you can use, provided of course that it is consumed in sensible amounts.

## Polyunsaturated Fats and Oils:

In sharp contrast to saturated and monounsaturated fats, the polyunsaturated fats in vegetable and seed oils are easily oxidised and they undergo further oxidation in a manufacturing process that also damages their molecular structure. This occurs because the seeds and nuts that are used to make the oils are heated to high temperatures, exposed to high pressures and mixed with chemicals and solvents during the manufacturing process. Consumption of such chemically altered oils disrupts our normal metabolism and provides a major source of free radicals. The richer the oil in polyunsaturated fatty acids and the longer it is exposed to heat, light and oxygen, the lower the quality of the oil becomes, the more free radicals in contains and the more damage it is capable of causing.

Because the flavour of poor quality highly oxidised oils can be masked by heavy seasoning, the lowest quality oils are often used in the manufacture of salad dressings and mayonnaise. Ironically, more often than not, these are presented as being the 'healthy' or 'lite' option. Even the premium priced cold-processed oils sold in health food stores, can also contain damaging free radicals because as soon as they are extracted and exposed to oxygen and light they begin to oxidise. Irrespective of whether they are cold pressed or heat extracted, heating any type of polyunsaturated vegetable oils to high temperatures to fry food will compound the problem. When any oil is heated, the rate of oxidation increases rapidly, doubling with every ten degrees centigrade rise in temperature, so the more the oil is heated the more free radicals are produced. Polyunsaturated oils come complete with their own supply of free radicals plus the free radicals that they have inherited from the manufacturing and cooking process. However, once they are inside our body they undergo a further process of peroxidation and this results in yet more free radicals. The fatty acid or 'lipid' peroxides that result from this have the potential to create an enormous amount of damage to our cells and blood vessels as well as cell DNA and as a consequence they put an ever increasing load on our body's need for antioxidants.

In a typical Western diet around 30% of a days calories come from polyunsaturated oils. This is an astonishingly high figure and research indicates that this amount is far too high. The best evidence suggests that the daily intake of polyunsaturates should be around 4% of the total number of calories. No one ever ate oils like this a hundred years ago because they simply did not exist. Where do the oils come from? Salad dressings, mayonnaise, fried foods, chips, fries, cakes, biscuits, processed foods. Its a long list and more often than not we are eating them without even realising it.

## Margarine, Shortening and 'Trans Fats'

### Is Margarine a healthier option than butter?

Well for years we have been told that it is. However, a process called 'hydrogenation' is used to convert polyunsaturated fats that are liquid at room temperature into Trans Fats that are solid at room temperature. In reality Trans Fats are Polyunsaturated Vegetable Oils (PUFA') in their worst possible form and they are found in just about all of the processed food we eat.

The manufacturing process of Hydrogenation is far from being a healthy process and not surprisingly the end result of the process is not a healthy product. Polyunsaturated oils that are already heavy in free radicals from the extraction process are mixed with a catalyst that is then subjected to hydrogen gas in a high pressure, high temperature reactor. Hence 'hydrogenated'. Emulsifiers and starch are then added to improve the consistency and the oil is again subjected to high temperatures in order to steam clean it and remove any unpleasant smells. Bleach, dyes and flavours are then added to make it look like and taste like butter. By the time margarine reaches your table it is a completely unnatural product and hardly the healthy food it is promoted as being! Trans fats are polyunsaturated vegetable oils in their worst possible form.

The high temperatures and chemicals used in the hydrogenation process not only create even more free radicals, they also transform the chemical structure of the oils that are used by changing the position of some of the hydrogen atoms. Hence the name trans fats. As it is almost impossible to remove all of the chemicals used in the manufacturing process, most of these trans fats contain small amounts of toxins as well as a load of free radicals. Because the trans fats mimic naturally occurring fats the body doesn't recognise them as being different and as a consequence they are not excreted. Instead, just like any other naturally occurring polyunsaturated fat they are incorporated into cell membranes where they wreak havoc, disrupting the cells metabolism and ultimately damaging or killing the cell. The end result is high levels of uric acid and inflammation at the site of the cell death, yet more free radicals and more pressure on our body's antioxidant defences, at a time when the body is being deprived of the raw materials it needs to make them. A strong correlation between hydrogenated fats and disease was observed as long ago as the 1940's but despite this, more than seventy years on, they are still being promoted as being the 'healthy' option.

Trans Fats in the form of margarine and shortening have the commercially pleasing property of being able to extend a products shelf life. They are also cheap. As a consequence they are widely used in manufactured and processed foods. Look on a label and you will see 'hydrogenated vegetable fat' as one of the ingredients. Margarine, vegetable shortening, non dairy creamers and non dairy whipped toppings all contain trans fats, as do most of the biscuits, cakes and 'junk' food in your local supermarket. As with the polyunsaturated oils from which they are derived, no one ever ate food like this years ago because it simply did not exist.

# When Iron Behaves Badly

## Its All About Balance

Sometimes, when we are overloaded with free radicals or when certain essential vitamins and minerals are in short supply, our body doesn't work quite as well as it should. We have talked about uric acid and Xanthine Oxidase, both of which can under certain conditions produce free radicals. Well, when the body has too much iron, the iron itself can also lead to the generation of free radicals.

Iron is essential for life. It is used in our blood to transport oxygen around our body. It is used in the conversion of sugar, fats and proteins into Adenosine Triphosphate (ATP), the store of energy that is inside all of our cells, and it is an essential constituent of one of the antioxidants our bodies make, catalase. However, as we saw earlier, despite its importance, too much iron can sometimes cause problems.

Because iron is so important to us it has a selective advantage when it competes with other metals and minerals like zinc, copper and manganese for absorption. As a consequence it is easy for us to become saturated with iron at the expense of other trace elements. Some of these trace elements play an important role in our body's own endogenous antioxidant defences and when this happens iron can cause antioxidant enzymes to malfunction by replacing the trace elements they need to make them work effectively. One of these is Superoxide Dismutase, an important antioxidant that is involved in the process of mopping up the superoxide free radicals produced when uric acid is made. Superoxide Dismutase needs zinc and copper, so when we are saturated with iron these are not available and there is not enough active Superoxide Dismutase and the superoxide radicals remain unchecked. Superoxide Dismutase is not the only endogenous antioxidant that high levels of iron can have an adverse effect on. While iron is needed for the antioxidant catalase, glutathione peroxidase and another antioxidant metallothionein both need copper, so when it is short supply because the body has absorbed iron in preference to copper, their effectiveness is also reduced.

The HEME and non HEME iron that we consume in our food is in the form of ions. These ions are 'positively' charged particles and they need something to attach themselves to in order to 'neutralise' this positive charge. When molecules of various proteins 'bind' to them they are neutralised. The terms 'liganded' or 'chelated' are used to describe this process. Both uric acid and Vitamin C have the ability to chelate and bind to iron as well as other metal ions. The anthocyanins and polyphenols that are present in some of the food we eat are also known to be able to do this. However, if the inactivation process is for some reason incomplete and the iron ions still retain their charge they can react and produce some of the body's most dangerous free radicals.

Superoxide and hydrogen peroxide free radicals are generated in the body through various processes. Under normal conditions these two free radicals rarely interact. However, in the presence of certain metal ions, particularly iron, a sequence of reactions can take place and this produces Hydroxyl radicals. Hydrogen peroxide produces the hydroxyl radical by removing an electron from the metal ion, but a sort of chain reaction then follows as the metal ion is regenerated by superoxide. It is then able to react with more hydrogen peroxide to produce yet more hydroxyl radicals.

Hydroxyl radicals have a very short life, they are highly reactive and they work at a localised level. This makes them very dangerous compounds that are known to damage DNA, cell membranes and amino acids. They can also react with hydrogen peroxide in another chain reaction that produces yet more free radicals, this time in the form of peroxyl radicals. Unlike superoxide radicals which can be rendered harmless by Superoxide Dismutase, these hydroxyl and peroxyl radicals can not be eliminated by any of the body's own antioxidant enzymes on their own. They need a hefty team of dietary antioxidants as well as our body's own endogenous antioxidants to work together to make them safe. This, combined with the lower levels of endogenous antioxidants caused by iron overload, means that they are a major source of cell damage and oxidative stress, both of which lead to increased levels of uric acid, inflammation and yet more free radicals.

# Cooking Methods

## Can cooking methods produce damaging substances?

One of the most intriguing aspects of the modern 'Western' diet is the high heat at which so much of our food is cooked. We fry food in fat or oil, we grill it, we BBQ it and we roast and bake it in hot ovens. The effect that these cooking methods have on our food is immense. None of the food we eat, irrespective of whether it is of animal or plant origin, is designed to withstand cooking at such high temperatures and as a consequence its nutritional content and chemical structure both suffer.

Why do we cook foods? Well, while some foods can be eaten in their raw, natural state, sometimes cooking is needed in order to:

- make food safe to eat by killing bacteria
- tenderise foods that would otherwise be tough and unpleasant to eat
- increase the time the food can be kept for
- increase the amount of nutrients or energy we are able to absorb from the food
- make the food easier to digest

Cooking also has the benefit of improving the taste and flavour of food and making it look more appetising.

### What are the consequences of cooking at high temperatures?

Nutritional research is only just starting to catch up with the consequences of our high temperature cooking methods and our addiction to 'browned', 'caramelised' and 'crisp' foods. From the previous section we know that when oils are heated they oxidise and produce free radicals; the higher the temperature the greater the number of free radicals. But this isn't the only thing that happens. Cooking at high temperatures, even in the absence of oil, can transform otherwise healthy foods into unhealthy compounds that can cause serious damage to our cells and the DNA within the cells. Heterocyclic amines (HCA's), and polycyclic aromatic hydrocarbons (PAH's), Acrylamide and Advanced Glycation End Products (AGE's) that are also called Glycotoxins, are just some of these compounds. When it comes to hyperuricemia and gout the compounds that are of most interest are the Advanced Glycation End products as these affect just about every type of cell in the body. They are also thought to be a major factor in some age related diseases and they are known to be linked to oxidative stress, insulin resistance and diabetes.

## What are AGE's and where do they come from?

AGE's come from two sources, our bodies and our food. Our bodies produce them as part of normal metabolism. Carbohydrates, irrespective of whether they are simple or complex, are metabolised into glucose and used by our body as a source of energy. However, a small amount of this glucose is glycated to form AGE's. As we get older AGE's are produced in greater numbers and they are also produced in greater numbers if we have higher than normal amounts of glucose in our blood. Scientists studying diabetes have known about the existence of AGE's for years. They have also known that simple sugars like fructose are glycated ten times faster than glucose. With the dramatic increase in the consumption of sugar, the number of people with high levels of blood sugar and as a consequence high levels of AGE's has increased dramatically over recent years.

Dietary AGE's form as food browns during cooking, primarily when foods high in protein or fat are subjected to high temperatures. When you fry a piece of steak or cook it under the grill you are creating a chemical reaction called a Maillard reaction. This occurs when some of the sugars, fats and proteins in the food react together when they are exposed to high temperatures. The end result are glycotoxins or AGE's. While cooking in dry heat produces the most AGE's, pasteurisation, smoking and microwaving all produce them. Because the beans from which they are made are roasted even coffee and chocolate contain them. The higher the roasting temperature and the longer the roasting time the more AGE's they contain. Any food that contains sugars, fats and proteins is fair game. One of the worrying things about AGE's is that for most of us the browning effect they come from enhances the flavour of food. As a consequence they increase our appetite and this encourages us to eat more. It is not surprising that the food manufacturing industry has taken this interesting characteristic on board and now adds sugar in various forms to certain foods in order to enhance their colour and flavour and entice us to eat more; biscuits, baked goods, ready meals and colas all contain them.

## Why should we worry about AGE's?

Once inside the body AGE's can damage cells, tissues and organs and this damage causes increased levels of uric acid and inflammation. They can also accelerate the general ageing process. The sulphated mucopolysaccharides that form part of the connective tissue that lubricates our joints are known to reduce and breakdown as we get older leaving residual calcium ions that have the potential to seed monosodium urate crystals. The total state of oxidative stress and age related damage is proportional to the dietary intake of AGE's and the consumption of sugar, in all its disguises. One other thing that we should really worry about is that high levels of AGE's are linked to decreased levels of testosterone, even in non diabetic men, and decreased levels of testosterone are linked to increased levels of uric acid and gout.

It is estimated that the standard American diet now contains about 10,000 and 16,000 kU of AGEs each day. This is three times higher than the safety limit advised by professional organisations. Most scientists agree that about ten per cent of the AGE's in our food are absorbed and of this 10%, it takes about three days for the body to excrete around a third of them. The remaining two thirds are not excreted. This means that as they slowly accumulate, there are plenty left hanging around in the body to cause trouble.

## What can we do about them?

Different foods produce different amounts of AGE's and different cooking methods also create different amounts. For example, if you fry, grill or roast a 90gram chicken breast it will generate between 4,000 to 9,000 units of AGE's. If you steam, boil or stew it it will produce about 1,000. As a general rule, because they contain less protein, vegetables produce fewer AGE's than animal based products. The more raw foods we eat the lower the number of AGE's. Interestingly, lemon juice and vinegar used as marinades decease the formation of AGE's. So by changing cooking methods, marinading your meat and fish in lemon juice or vinegar and eating less animal protein we can reduce the amount of AGE's we are exposing our bodies to.

### Can cooking methods produce damaging substances?

Yes, without doubt they can. While they are not themselves free radicals, AGE's damage cells and this damage increases levels of uric acid, gives rise to inflammation and this increases the load of free radicals the body has to cope with. High levels of AGE's are known to be linked to oxidative stress, insulin resistance, diabetes and reduced levels of testosterone all of which puts more pressure on our body's antioxidant defence systems.

### What about the Maori?

They ate fish, birds, eggs and vegetables and they cooked their food by boiling it or wrapping it in leaves and steaming it in a pit in the ground. They had no means of frying or roasting and the only oil they had was extracted by crushing the seeds of a native flax plant between stones. Their problems began when they not only changed their diet, they also changed their cooking methods and began using an oven and a frying pan.

## What About Alcohol?

### Is there a link between the consumption of alcohol and hyperuricemia?

When it comes to hyperuricemia and gout the consumption of alcohol is always a hot topic. Man has consumed alcohol in various forms for thousands of years. Even primitive man unknowingly consumed it when he ate fruit that was partially fermented. Our bodies also make small amounts of alcohol as part of normal daily living. However, once man became urbanised and was unable to safely drink water from streams and wells the brewing of beer made water safe. While wine was the drink of the rich and privileged, beer was the every day drink for all classes of people. Men, women and even children consumed beer and it was often consumed in quantities that to us are astounding. There is plenty of documentary evidence to support this. Notwithstanding that modern beer, at between 3% and 5%, is much stronger than the 1% to 2% 'small beer' that was consumed then, when drunk in large quantities it still amounts to a lot of alcohol. Records show that in Coventry in the 16th Century in England, the average person consumed about 17 pints of ale a week, six times more than the average consumption today. The household records of a 17th Century English stately home show that a groom, who incidentally rose at 5am and went to bed at 9pm, was given;

".... beer and bread for his breakfast at 8am, bread, cheese and beer for his lunch at mid day and bacon, beans and beer for his supper at 7pm ....."

While these household records do not state how much beer was given with each meal the records of the British armed services do. In addition to their rum and lime juice ration, British sailors received a ration of a gallon, 8 pints, of beer a day. Soldiers each received two thirds of a gallon. As a sailor's beer was usually brewed on board ship we know little about its alcohol content. We do however know about a soldiers' beer. This was in fact a 'porter' and at 6% this was definitely not a 'small beer'.

It is clear that in the past beer was consumed in quantities that are far in excess of today's guidelines. Yes, the life expectancy of the ordinary man then was much shorter, yet people then were far healthier than they are now. Hyperuricemia and gout was the disease of the wealthy, not the ordinary man. Almost all epidemiological studies find an association between alcohol, gout and healthy 'non drinking' control groups, but some scientists think that the link is not proven. The exact incidence of alcohol induced gout and hyperuricemia still remains unknown. What is known however is that beer drinkers are more likely to have gout than people who drink spirits and people who drink moderate amounts of red wine interestingly appear to have no increased risk of gout at all.

There is no doubt that there is some form of link between alcohol consumption and gout but what is the link? Well one of the interesting things about alcohol is the way in which it is consumed; different types of alcohol are consumed by different groups of people in different ways. Wine tends to be consumed with a meal that is in dietary terms relatively healthy, whereas beer tends to be consumed either on its own or accompanied by snacks that are often far from healthy. As a population, wine drinkers could simply be healthier, eat better quality foods or simply overall consume less alcohol.

Alcohol can induce hyperuricemia in a number of different ways:-

- All alcoholic drinks, irrespective of whether they are beer, lager, wine or spirits contain ethanol and ethanol is metabolised by the liver in exactly the same way as fructose. So when you consume alcohol you are effectively consuming fat. In addition, most alcoholic drinks also contain sugar in some shape or form and sugar provides unwanted calories that can ultimately end up as fat. As an example, beer contains a sugar called maltose. In a pint of beer there are about 30 grams of maltose and this means a pint of beer contains around 350 kcals. Red wine however contains very little sugar so one 125ml glass of red wine contains only around 100 calories.
- Irrespective of whether it is in the form of beer, lager, wine or spirits, alcohol is a diuretic and diuretics increase the amount of water we excrete. As a consequence when alcohol is consumed in quantity it can lead to dehydration and dehydration can potentially trigger an attack of gout.
- When consumed in large amounts over a short space of time lactic acid is produced as the alcohol is metabolised. The lactic acid can reduce the amount of uric acid excreted by the kidneys.
- Alcohol increases the absorption of iron and as we know, iron stimulates Xanthine Oxidase and the production of uric acid. High levels of iron are also linked to insulin resistance and diabetes, both of which reduce the amount of uric acid excreted.

- Alcohol induces increased levels of iron ions that are not bound to various proteins and, as described previously, this contributes to the formation of dangerous hydroxyl radicals.

As well as promoting the generation of free radicals and Reactive Oxygen Species, alcohol also interferes with the body's normal antioxidant defence mechanisms by stripping the body of some of its Vitamin C as well as some of the essential nutrients it needs to make its own endogenous antioxidants. Zinc is of particular interest here as alcohol not only increases the amount of zinc that is excreted, it also reduces the amount of zinc that is absorbed from food. So consuming alcohol on a regular basis, especially if it is consumed in relatively large amounts, can over time lead to low levels of zinc or in extreme cases zinc deficiency. One of our body's endogenous antioxidants that plays a key role in mopping up superoxide is Superoxide Dismutase. As this is a zinc based antioxidant low levels of zinc could reduce the amount of Superoxide Dismutase the body is able to make and hence directly lead to increased oxidative stress and from this hyperuricemia. The bottom line is that alcohol scores twice. First by increasing the free radical load your body is subjected to and then by reducing your body's ability to cope with the increased load.

As with antioxidants and free radicals, all sources of alcohol are not created equal. Red wine appears to have very little effect on hyperuricemia. Because of the tannins and polyphenols that it contains, red wine actually slows down the absorption of non HEME iron, even though it actually contains moderate amounts of this type of iron. When consumed as part of a meal it slows down the digestion of the meal and this results in more stable blood glucose levels. Because of this, red wine is the key element in what is often described as the 'French Paradox'; the consumption of a rich and potentially unhealthy diet that appears to be made healthy by the inclusion of moderate amounts of red wine. How can red wine make an unhealthy diet healthy? It contains a lot of antioxidants, polyphenols, Resveratrol and quercetin are just some of the them and in some way they appear to balance things out.

So where does this fit into the stereotypical historical view of the gout sufferer? They were the only people who could afford to drink wine and this should in theory have been of benefit to them. We can only assume that the way the wine was made and stored and the vessels from which it was consumed must have played their part.

The consumption of beer has for years been a complete 'no - no' when it comes to gout. But no one is able to provide a convincing reason why it is so much worse than wine or all of the other different types of alcohol. Even when a 'low purine diet' is discounted as an effective way of managing gout, the reason why beer is 'bad' is that it contains the purine Guanosine and Guanosine is one of the purines from which uric acid is made. Confusing.

Well, I have another theory about why beer is bad for gout and I think it is quite convincing. Firstly, like red wine beer contains iron. Around 1.2mg in a pint. However, unlike red wine it does not contain anything that inhibits the absorption of the iron so the iron in the beer simply adds to the daily iron load.

Secondly, beer contains lactic acid because lactic acid is produced when beer is brewed. Lactic acid is also produced when alcohol is metabolised, so beer is scoring twice. As we know, lactic acid reduces the amount of uric acid the kidney's excrete, but it also creates a sudden short term 'spike' in the pH of the blood that increases its acidity and this can increase the number of calcium ions present and hence seed the formation of uric acid crystals.

Last but not least, beer is made from malted barley and barley contains both sugar and protein. When barley is malted it is exposed to high temperatures. As with any type of heat process this produces AGE's, in this case the AGE's are in the form of melanoidins. These melanoidins give the beer its characteristic colour and flavour. The longer the malting process and the higher the temperature, the darker the beer and the higher its AGE content. If the malting process wasn't enough, beer is boiled when it is 'mashed', often for quite a long time and this creates yet more AGE's. The AGE's in beer have exactly the same damaging effect as any other AGEs, leading over time to cell damage, inflammation, insulin resistance, reduced levels of testosterone and ultimately increased levels of uric acid.

When you look at the evidence, alcohol is not a sensible choice if you suffer from hyperuricemia or gout. Apart from contributing to hyperuricemia and potentially triggering a gout flare, it also contains a lot of calories and carrying extra weight will serve only to make a bad situation worse. More important though is the simple fact that alcohol weakens your will power, so once you have had one drink it is easy to have another. Then before you know it a little demon takes over and you start 'snacking' as well, usually on the type of junk food that is not good for you.

So if you suffer from gout the best advice is to stop drinking completely for at least three months. If you do not want to stop drinking or you feel unable to, make sure that you drink plenty of water, preferably filtered water, and keep yourself well hydrated. If you do stop drinking, once you have been gout free for several months, then maybe you can experiment and find out if you can tolerate a glass of red wine or a small beer. However, there is no 'one size fits all solution' so the management of alcohol consumption will always remain a personal matter.

## What about the Maori?

They had no alcohol until the European settlers came and they only started consuming alcohol in significant quantity, in particular beer, once they became urbanised. With their genetic predisposition for gout, alcohol combined with the changes to their diet, lifestyle and cooking methods means that they now have one of the highest levels of gout in the world.

# Acidic & Inflammatory Food

## Food That Is 'Acidic'

- Is there a link between foods that are acidic and Hyperuricemia?
- Is it true that the food and drink we consume causes our blood and our bodies to become more alkaline or acidic?

Not strictly speaking, but there is an indirect link to gout. When you eat and drink the end products of digestion and the assimilation of the nutrients in the food and drink results in either an overall acid or alkaline effect. Because our body needs to maintain a pH of between 7.35 and 7.45, which is slightly alkaline, it uses its natural buffer systems to regulate the pH. Under normal circumstances this works fine but if you spend years eating a diet that is highly acidic these buffers ultimately become exhausted and the body has to call on its reserves, in particular its calcium phosphate reserves. When this happens it heads in the direction of our bones, joints and teeth and takes small amounts of calcium phosphate from them. In the process of doing this the concentration of calcium ions in the blood increases and this increases the risk of monosodium urate crystals 'seeding' around the ions and triggering an attack of gout. Its a process similar to what happens when there are sudden short term 'spikes' in pH due to lactic acid.

So which foods have an alkaline forming effect and which have an acid forming effect? Well most wheat grains, animal products, sugar, alcohol and highly processed foods have an acid forming effect and generally speaking most vegetables, fruit and unprocessed foods have an alkaline forming effect. Compared to vegetarians, people who eat animal protein, particularly in the form of meat, lose between two and four times the amount of calcium. The larger the amount of animal protein consumed the greater the loss of calcium.

Unfortunately vegetables, fruit and unprocessed foods are in short supply in the typical Western diet. Ideally you need to eat slightly more alkaline forming foods than acid forming foods in order to have a net effect that matches the body's normal pH. This will then reduce the pressure on the buffer systems.

## Foods That Are Inflammatory?

Today there is a growing consensus among medical professionals that inflammation plays a major role in many of the chronic diseases of the Western World and all of these are on the increase. Irrespective of whether there is a cause and effect relationship there is no doubt that inflammation provides a common link. While many are content to treat these diseases with drugs, more and more medical professionals are beginning to accept that treating the underlying cause of the inflammation would be a better long-term solution.

When our bodies metabolise the food we eat some of the nutrients in it are used to produce substances called prostaglandins. These prostaglandins can be either pro-inflammatory, in other words they create inflammation or increase a state of inflammation that already exists, or they can be anti-inflammatory and calm down or reduce inflammation. Imbalances in your diet can lead to excessive amounts of inflammatory prostaglandins being produced.

Gout is a form of inflammatory arthritis. So if you have gout your body is in a state of chronic systemic inflammation. Any pro inflammatory food you consume will simply fuel this inflammation. Refined grains, animal products, processed meats, sugar, polyunsaturated vegetable oils, hydrogenated oils in the form of trans fats, soft drinks and foods that are fried and cooked at high temperatures, are on most people's menus and these are all inflammatory. In contrast anti-inflammatory foods like wholegrains, beans and pulses, nuts and seeds, fresh fruit and vegetables, herbs and spices and fish form a very small part of a typical Western diet.

Probably the two most important foods that are fuelling inflammation are polyunsaturated vegetable oils and sugar, in all their forms and disguises. Iron rich foods come in a close third. Notwithstanding that the consumption of sugar has increased enormously over the last hundred years, it is the polyunsaturated vegetable oils that are the most interesting as they are effectively a new kid on the block and its a pretty unruly kid at that.

As discussed earlier unsaturated fatty acids primarily come in two groups, Omega-3 and Omega-6. Each of these groups has a 'parent' from which all of the fatty acids in the group are made. In the case of the Omega-3 group this is ALA or alpha linoleic acid and in the case of the Omega-6 group this is LA or linoleic acid. Because the body is unable to make these 'parents' and they have to come from our food they are Essential Fatty Acids or EFA's. Of the two Omega-3 is by far the most important in terms of being beneficial to our health. Why? Because Omega-3 fatty acids suppress inflammation and Omega-6 fatty acids promote it. Omega-3 fats are found abundantly in seafood, nuts and a few seeds like flax. To a lesser extent they are also found in meat, dairy products and green vegetables. Omega-6 fats occur naturally in small amounts in nuts and seeds but they are abundant in manufactured vegetable oils and hydrogenated trans fats, foods that have been around for less than a hundred years.

In the good old days when Omega-3 and Omega-6 fats were obtained naturally from food that was unprocessed things were quite well balanced. We were consuming them in a ratio of between one Omega-3 to one Omega-6 or at most one Omega-3 to four Omega-6. With the advent of polyunsaturated vegetable oils this ratio changed dramatically. Because we consume so much vegetable oil and hydrogenated vegetable oil in the form of trans fats, many of us now consume up to twenty or thirty times more Omega-6 than Omega-3 and this creates a highly inflammatory environment. This has major consequences when added to the other pro-inflammatory foods we are consuming. Combined with the Western diet of over refined carbohydrates, sugar and processed foods it simply fuels the inflammation that these are also creating.

## Saturated Fats and Inflammation

In researching hyperuricemia and the causes of gout, I have read over and over again that 'saturated fat' increases the amount of uric acid we have as well as reducing the amount of uric acid that is excreted. Despite making a major effort I have not succeeded in finding the scientific evidence or the source of this statement. It appears to be another of the 'gout diet myths'. The only link I can find is that saturated fat contains among other things Arachidonic Acid (AA), an Omega 6 fat that is a precursor of pro-inflammatory hormones. We know that all animal proteins and fats are categorised as generally being 'inflammatory' foods. However, vegetable oils and trans fats contain vastly more Omega 6 fats than the saturated fat found in butter, cheese, eggs and meat. So the real culprit appears to be the vegetable oils we consume in such large amounts and not the saturated fats everyone seems to talk about.

## What about the quality of the food we eat?

I have thought long and hard about including this section as I have no wish to sound 'cranky'. However, the quality of the food we eat is highly relevant, especially when it comes to inflammation.

We know that the amount of meat we are eating has on average doubled over the last 50 years and that we are consuming far more animal protein than we need to, but what about the quality of the meat we eat? Is it better or worse than it was 50 or 60 years ago? In view of the intensive farming methods now being used it is hardly surprising that quality has fallen dramatically. Most commercially produced meat and poultry is from animals reared in sheds or pens and even fish is now farmed in large quantities. Instead of feeding on grass, cattle are now fed on grain, pigs no longer root around fields eating their natural omnivorous diet and chickens no longer scratch around eating whatever they can find. As a consequence the nutritional content of the meat, fish and eggs from industrially reared animals is very different to the meat, fish and eggs from animals living in their natural environment.

The idiom '*You are what you eat*' certainly holds true here. When you look at farmed salmon, the ratio of Omega-3 to Omega-6 fats is very different to the ratio of fats found in wild salmon. Organic free range eggs have a much healthier Omega-3 to Omega-6 ratio than eggs from battery hens, even when the hens are fed on fish meal so that they lay 'Omega-3 enhanced' eggs . While the difference in overall fat content of meat from intensively reared and grass fed is usually only about 5%, the difference in the type of fat in these animals is very significant. Depending on breed, grass fed beef has between 2 and 5 times the amount of Omega 3 than grain fed beef. It also has more conjugated linoleic acid and considerably more antioxidants, vitamins and minerals. While grass fed beef has more iron and zinc than grain fed beef, it has much lower levels of antibiotics and artificial hormones and this more than compensates for the extra iron.

## Where does this fit in with hyperuricemia and gout.

Put simply the over consumption of pro-inflammatory foods and the under consumption of anti-inflammatory foods is putting an enormous strain on our immune system and effectively 'wearing us out'. It is most definitely not making a positive contribution to our health.

## Does history support the concept that we are what we eat?

Well historically gout was the 'disease of kings', a disease that only afflicted the rich, the privileged and the 'men of the cloth'.

Only the rich could afford to eat flour that was in any way refined and 'white'. As you went down through the social scale less wheat and more rye and oatmeal was consumed and the coarser and less refined this 'flour' became. By the time you got to the peasants, the really poor, they couldn't afford flour at all. They ate a sort of meal made from ground up beans or pulses.

The rich ate meat and they ate it in large amounts. The less money you had the less meat and animal protein you consumed. When you got to the poor they ate hardly any. They lived almost exclusively on vegetables. Any animals they had were far too valuable in providing milk or eggs for them to be eaten.

Only the rich roasted their food. They roasted it on spits at a high temperature in front of an open fire The poor boiled or stewed their food. They used a single large pot that was hung over the fire. Ovens and cooking ranges only became widely available to the middle and upper classes in early Victorian times. The poor continued to use the 'stew pot' until well into the 19th Century.

Historically carbohydrates generally were in short supply. There were no potatoes and there was no rice. The carbohydrates that were available were all complex and unrefined. Sugar was an extremely expensive luxury, as was honey, and only the very rich could afford to buy it. With the exception of small amounts of fruit that could be dried or stored, fruit was seasonal. Only the rich could afford the sugar or honey needed to preserve it.

Interestingly the monks had gout and in most orders they ate a predominantly vegetarian diet. But they also lived very austere lives and their frequent prayers meant that they had heavily disrupted short sleep cycles. They also spent a lot of time kneeling on cold stone floors.

In the homes of the rich and wealthy as well as in the monasteries, pewter was used for tableware and cooking utensils. Lead could easily have leached into their food, slowly accumulated in their systems and impaired the way their kidneys worked.

Alcohol. Well this is a paradox. Beer or ale was consumed by all, the poorer classes consuming the most, and it was consumed in amounts that to us are astoundingly high. Spirits as such were extremely rare. Paradoxically it was the rich who drank wine and they were the people suffering from gout, but in those days wine was made in lead lined containers and often preserved and sweetened with lead acetate. Could the mead the monks are reputed to have brewed from honey have anything to do with their gout? It would have contained large amounts of residual sugar as well as lead that was leached from the pots in which it was made.

## Are we really what we eat?

Well I think the evidence is over whelming. Polyunsaturated vegetable oils, trans fats, too much iron, over refined carbohydrates, and this includes sugar in all its disguises, alcohol, a lack of antioxidants and changed cooking methods are all taking their toll. I believe that we really are what we eat. In fact I am convinced that we are and that diet, cooking methods and lifestyle are major factors in the dramatic increase in not only gout but also many of the other chronic diseases that are becoming so prevalent in the Western World. This means that changes to our diet and the way in which we cook the food we eat and live our daily lives can have only a positive impact on our health.

CHAPTER 9

# Where Did It All Go Wrong?

In less than 100 years the general state of health of the western world has deteriorated rapidly and it is continuing to do so at an alarming rate. In 1980 150 million people were thought to be suffering from diabetes. Today this figure is nearer to 360 million. Even among children metabolic syndrome and obesity is close to becoming an epidemic. If we look back into even recent history it is clear that both our lifestyle and our diet have changed dramatically. Lack of exercise, over refined carbohydrates, sugar, junk food and TV diners are all taking their toll on our health.

Whether we like it or not, the bottom line is that we all eat too much. We simply eat more than our bodies need and most of us are unaware that we are doing this because large amounts of sugar and the wrong sort of fat are hidden in our food. We are also eating too much of the wrong foods. Foods that are actually damaging our health. We have been fed misinformation and in effect conned by big business and advertising into believing that some foods are good for us when in fact they are not. The triumph of partially hydrogenated vegetable fats as being a healthier option than butter is a classical example of this. I for one really did believe that vegetable oils and margarine were a healthier option than saturated fats.

We all lead busy lives and as a consequence quick meals are sometimes a necessity. For most of us cooking and preparing food is seen as a chore. Many of us would prefer to watch TV or read a book than cook. I think the problem really started when we began to 'manufacture' food, and I mean 'manufacture' in the widest sense of the word. The intensive farming of beef and poultry is just another type of manufacturing. When we started manufacturing food it became available in large quantities at a price that ordinary people could afford. At the same time it became easy for us to eat food that would otherwise take a long time to prepare and cook. Luxury foods like biscuits, cookies, cakes, chips, fries, mayonnaise and processed meats became widely available, so the ordinary man was able to eat more and at the same time also adopt some of the eating habits of the rich. Sixty years ago you were lucky if you ate meat once a week. Now many people eat it every day, sometimes at every meal. How often do you eat chicken or turkey? Well sixty years ago chicken and turkey were luxury foods. They were the preserve of the wealthy. The ordinary man was lucky if he ate them once a year at Christmas or Thanksgiving, now we can eat them any time we want.

We know that in the early 1920's average uric acid levels across the American population were around 3.5 mg/dl. In the past 90 years they have risen to between 4.0 and 5.5mg/dl. An enormous increase. How many 'manufactured' foods were available in 1920? No where near the number there are today. When did they first appear on the scene? Well we know that sugar goes back a very long way. But what about breakfast cereals. They were first packaged as a wholegrain health food in the late 1800's, but by the 1920's they began to evolve into the sugar coated flakes, hoops and puffs that we know today. Why did we change our eating habits and adopt manufactured and processed foods as part of our daily diet so quickly? The answer to this would fill volumes. What we do know is that many of the manufactured foods that have come onto the scene since the early 1900's are a smoking gun when it comes to gout, hyperuricemia and other chronic diseases. Over refined carbohydrates, sugar, polyunsaturated vegetable oils, trans fats and processed meats are most certainly not contributing positively to the health of the nation.

When it comes to the food industry, it is very difficult not to become political. However, it is an undeniable fact that food manufacturing is now big business, with companies spending billions of dollars a year on aggressive advertising that is geared to preserving their bottom line profits and not the health and well being of the people consuming the food they make.

Manufactured foods bring with them a whole raft of problems not least of which is the addition of compounds that are designed to enhance their appearance and extend their shelf life. Most food processing takes out many of the good things and adds back in a lot of bad things. Manufactured and processed foods are generally speaking impoverished products. Because of this our diet contains too many calories that have been stripped of most of the essential trace nutrients necessary for their proper assimilation. The high-speed milling of grains such as wheat, rice, and corn results in the reduction or removal of more than twenty nutrients, including some essential fatty acids and the majority of their minerals and trace elements. In order to make your body's internally produced antioxidant team you need these minerals and trace elements. Without these antioxidants free radicals are not neutralised and oxidative stress develops at an ever-increasing rate.

Like many things in life food can be addictive and manufactured and processed foods really are addictive, the food manufacturers have made sure of that. Dietary habits are just that, habits, and like all habits they can be changed. However, urging someone to change the eating habits of a lifetime is no easy task. It is a fact that less than 20% of patients seeking medical advice are prepared to make substantial lifestyle and dietary changes. However, in the management of hyperuricemia and gout, dietary and lifestyle changes are crucially important. If you suffer from gout your body is not functioning properly and in order to get it back into proper working order, the essential first step towards leading a gout free life, you need a long term solution. There is no magic cure or silver bullet.

For years the gout sufferer has been told that cherry juice, apple cider vinegar, bicarbonate of soda, red cabbage, tablets of green tea and special food supplements were the wonder foods that would cure their gout. The sad reality is that you cannot rectify a diet that is overloaded with the wrong foods and completely lacking in the essential vitamins, minerals and antioxidants it so desperately needs by simply taking a one off cure. We need to look at the 'big picture' and correct the underlying causes of gout and hyperuricemia.

## What is The New Gout Diet?

Well its not a diet in the typical meaning of the word as there are no meal plans and there is no calorie counting. It is more of an eating, cooking and food selection programme that is designed to help you eat wisely. It is a set of guidelines as opposed to a set of strict rules. Its all about making a switch from the foods that can cause gout to the foods that will restore your body's natural balance and set you on the road to leading a gout free life. The occasional mishap won't spell doom. Its what you do most of the time, not what you do some of the time that matters and, unlike some rigidly restrictive gout diets, it does not take the fun out of eating. You don't have to give up eggs and butter or any of the other foods high in purines that have for so long been unjustly given a bad press. Notwithstanding this, its important to understand that your diet is going to change and for some this change could be significant. Eventually you are likely to be eating in a very different way to the way you are eating now.

### How is this achieved?

- By reducing your consumption of foods that increase levels of insulin. In other words refined carbohydrates and sugar. By doing this you can begin to get your insulin sensitivity under control.
- Reducing the load of free radicals that your body has to contend with. This means not only consuming less of the foods that contain large amounts of free radicals, it also means consuming less of the foods that create too many free radicals when they are metabolised.
- Optimising the amount of antioxidants you consume in your food as well as the trace elements, vitamins, minerals and fats your body needs to make its own antioxidants.
- Using less oxidising and damage causing cooking methods
- Reducing your consumption of acid forming foods and increasing your consumption of alkaline forming foods as this will reduce the load on your body's phosphate buffers and reduce the chance of crystals of uric acid being formed.

- Reducing your consumption of pro-inflammatory foods, increasing your consumption of anti-inflammatory foods and eating an anti-inflammatory diet.

  This probably sounds like quite a challenge. Put simply, the new gout diet is all about going 'Back to Basics' and unless you can find a safe and reliable source of healthy manufactured foods this means cooking. Can't cook, won't cook, don't know how to cook? It is not as hard as you think. After all its only over the last fifty to sixty years that we stopped cooking. Taking back control of cooking could well be the single most important step you take on the road to recovery. Reclaiming cooking will provide you with healthier food, it will make you self reliant and it will open a door to a more enjoyable and nourishing life.

CHAPTER 10

# It's Goodbye To Gout

## The New Gout Diet

For many years a major supermarket chain in the UK has been using the advertising slogan

'Every little helps'

In their case they are saying that every penny counts towards the total amount you will save when you shop in their store. When it comes to gout and a diet that will enable you to live gout free every vitamin, mineral, antioxidant and micro nutrient, no matter how small, will contribute towards the well balanced diet that your body needs. If you are reading this you are one of the 20% of gout sufferers who are prepared to make, or at least think about making some major changes to your diet and lifestyle. The purpose of this book is to inform you and provide you with the information that will help you make these changes. But first a word about lifestyle.

### Being over weight:

When it comes to gout weight is a big factor. A Body Mass Index, BMI, above normal is one of the most important risk factors for gout. Whether increased weight is a 'lifestyle' issue that is linked to the consumption of sugar and over refined carbohydrates, lack of exercise or simply consuming more calories than your body needs is not clear. One thing is certain though, losing weight will have a positive impact, not least because it will reduce the general state of inflammation that your body is in and take some of the pressure off of your swollen and painful joints.

We each have our own individual preferences for a balance of different foods; meat and fish, fruits and vegetables, potatoes, rice and pasta. Food transforms us. It provides the building blocks for the amazing body that we live in. As we age we gain weight. The average American is thought to gain around one pound a year between the age of twenty and seventy. However, it appears that calories are not quite equal when it comes to their ability to make us gain weight. Some people continue to be over weight while eating less than 1,000 calories a day. Others stay slim even when eating five times this amount. While genetics do come into play here, it is important to remember that insulin and insulin resistance both play a major part in whether or not we gain weight and also how we lose it.

If you suffer from gout and you have a high BMI losing weight is one of the best things you can do. There are many types of 'diets', some are high in protein and low in carbohydrate, some are low in protein and high in carbohydrate, others are somewhere in between and focus on low GI complex carbohydrates which trigger less of a surge in the release of insulin. Today the conventional Western diet has about 75% of its calories coming from carbohydrate. It also has an upside down balance of Omega 3 and Omega 6 essential fatty acids and this leads to inflammation. There is strong evidence that for the gout sufferer a calorie restricted diet of around 1,600 calories a day that is high in fibre, low in carbohydrates and high in protein and unsaturated fat from fish, nuts and olive oil, can be beneficial.

## What about crash dieting?

Don't even think about it. Starvation, 'feast and fast' crash dieting and fad diets will really upset your body's metabolism and the end result will be that your body produces ketones and that you become stressed. The ketones will compete with uric acid for excretion by your kidneys and your uric acid levels will increase, potentially triggering a gout attack.

## Exercise

Or to be more precise the lack of it! How much exercise do you get each day? For the vast majority of us the answer is, 'not a lot'. Regular exercise will help with insulin sensitivity and go some way to reducing the negative effects that high levels of insulin is having on your uric acid levels. Regular exercise also helps by boosting your immune system and this will have a positive effect on the level of oxidative stress in your body.

When you exercise your body produces some very powerful hormones; endorphins, serotonin and dopamine. At the same time the level of stress hormones like Cortisol are reduced. Endorphins are the body's natural 'feel good' factor. When they are released through exercise they work together to make you feel good, your mood is boosted and you feel a general state of well being. You feel happy afterwards. However, do not delude yourself, you can not exercise yourself out of a bad diet.

A change to your diet goes hand and hand with exercise. What sort of exercise. Well it doesn't have to be anything too strenuous, you certainly don't need to join a gym. In fact joining a gym is probably the last thing you should do. Strenuous exercise can potentially lead to trauma that triggers a gout flare and it can also lead to 'spikes' of lactic acid and, as we know, this can reduce the amount of uric acid your body excretes and potentially seed crystals of uric acid. The 'have got to go to the gym' or 'go for a run' syndrome will also provide yet another stress factor that brings with it another set of adverse consequences. Mild, gentle exercise has no appreciable effect on lactic acid and just ten minutes each day can improve your mood. Try using the stairs instead of the lift or the escalator more often. Walking is great. Just half an hour four or five times a week will improve your health dramatically.

So what are the good things to eat, what are the 'not quite so good' and what are the bad things?

Unfortunately the 'Bad' list is quite long! Why? Well it contains just about all of the foods the food technologists have created over the last eighty to ninety years and they are the foods many of us eat nearly every day. So if the bad list is long, maybe we should start with the good list and you will pleased to hear that it is longer than you think! But first, a general word about allergies.

## A general word about allergies.

Gout is a form of inflammatory arthritis so if you suffer from gout your body is in a state of inflammation. One of the objectives of a gout diet is to reduce that inflammation. Without wishing to sound cranky, one of the reasons you have gout could be that you are 'intolerant' of some of the foods you consume on a regular basis and as a consequence they are contributing to a state of systemic inflammation; wheat gluten, eggs, soy, dairy and some types of nuts, especially peanuts, are known allergens. Lactose intolerance in particular is far more common than we realise.

Figures vary but between 5% and 20% of people of Caucasian descent have a level of lactose intolerance. Around 35% of the South Sea Islanders descended from the Taiwanese Aboriginals have the problem. In people of African decent the figure rises to between 65% and 75%, while in some Asian populations the figures is as high as 90%.

If you suspect that you are sensitive to a specific food or group of foods try eliminating it for at least two weeks. Listen to your body and see if symptoms like lethargy, headaches, flatulence or bloating subside. Tedious and time consuming it may be but its worth it in the long term.

# The Good, The 'Not Quite So Good' and The Bad

## The Good:

- Vegetables, Pulses and Fruit
- Fish, especially oily cold water fish
- Nuts and Seeds
- Tea, White, Green and Oolong
- Herbs and Spices
- Dairy Products, especially low fat dairy products
- Eggs
- Tofu, Soya Bean Curd and Tempeh
- Butter and Saturated Fats
- Olive Oil
- Chocolate and Cocoa
- Water, good old fashioned 'Adams' Ale'

## The 'Not Quite So Good':

- Whole Grains;
- Oatmeal, Quinoa, Millet, Buckwheat, Bulgar Wheat, Spelt and Barley
- Pasta
- Rice and Rice Noodles
- The Humble Potato
- Coffee

## The Bad:

- Refined Carbohydrates
- Sugar and High Fructose Corn Syrup
- Polyunsaturated Vegetable Oils and Trans Fats
- Alcohol; Beer, Lager, Cider, Wine and Spirits
- Food that contains iron
- Cooking Methods that fry, grill and roast at high temperatures
- Fruit juice and smoothies.

# The Good

## Vegetables, Pulses and Fruit

**Why?**

Vegetables and fruit are simply packed full of goodness and they taste great. They contain vitamins, minerals, trace elements and large amounts of antioxidants. As a general rule they are alkaline and many have anti-inflammatory properties. Flavonoids and bioflavonoids, phytonutrients, anthocyanins, carotenes, quercetin, resveratrol are just some of a long list of health giving compounds that fruit and vegetables contain. You name it they've got it and because they are so colourful they look wonderful on your plate.

Ever wondered why fruit and vegetables are so colourful? Flavonoids and bioflavonoids, their old name was tannins, and lycopene are compounds that give vegetables and fruit, grains, leaves and flowers their colour. Colours range from reds and orange to purple, mauve and blue. These compounds protect the plants from ultra violet light, disease and predators. The general rule is the brighter and stronger the colour, the greater the health benefits.

Green leafy vegetables, celery, beans, sweet potatoes, squashes, peppers, aubergines, pumpkins, berries, apples, oranges, lemons and limes. The list of vegetables and fruit that are available for us to eat is massive. We are wired to eat them and whether you eat them raw or cooked, they should form a major part of your gout diet. At least five portions of fruit and vegetables a day is really good advice.

Tomatoes are particularly interesting vegetables as they break all of the rules about cooking. Whereas with most vegetables their nutritional content, especially Vitamin C and other antioxidants, is damaged by cooking, tomatoes are not. The intense vibrant colour of a tomato is due to a very powerful antioxidant called lycopene that it contains. Lycopene is the major carotenoid found in red fruit and vegetables. Instead of being damaged or destroyed by cooking lycopene actually becomes more bio-available and this makes tomatoes in any shape or form a very valuable source of antioxidants. But take note. Some people can have an adverse reaction to tomatoes and other members of what is called "the nightshade" family of plants. Aubergines (egg plants), peppers and potatoes are also in this group. The adverse reaction is probably due to a substance called solanine that these vegetables contain. Some people think that tomatoes can actually trigger an attack of gout so take care.

Pulses are a particularly valuable vegetable as they are low in carbohydrate but high in protein and fibre. Red and black beans, chick peas, butter beans, borlotti beans, haricot beans, lentils and dried split peas are the staple food of millions of people around the world.

#### How?

Eat as many vegetables as you want. They are on 'free issue' on a gout diet. Be a bit careful about grapes and apples, fruits that contain a lot of fructose. In reality unless you eat your way through a several hundred grams of grapes or an awful lot of apples you are unlikely to be eating enough during a day to cause any real problems in terms of excess fructose consumption. We need to remember that the antioxidants in food exists first and foremost to protect the food itself from damage. So the whole food, often including its skin, is often more powerful than individual isolated elements. Eat your vegetables raw as a salad, steamed, braised, baked or stir fried very quickly at not too high a heat, more lightly sautéed than fried. The less you cook them the more nutritious the vegetables are. In reality you cannot eat too many vegetables. Whatever you do don't over cook them, eat them a little 'al dente'. If you do over cook them they will loose a lot of their goodness.

Use beans and pulses instead of potatoes, rice and pasta. Why? Because 100 grams of red beans contains only 8 grams of carbohydrate, which is far lower than the 80 grams in the same amount of rice and they are also a valuable source of protein and fibre. Puréed and mixed with herbs and tahini vegetables make greats dips and spreads Try snacking on celery and sticks of carrot, cucumber and sliced red and green peppers. Our grand children call them 'thunder sticks' because they go crunch when you eat them.

Our palettes vary enormously and to some people some vegetables have a highly unpleasant 'sulphur' taste. Try adding a small amount of chopped basil or basil pesto after they are cooked, it seems to mask the sulphur taste. This is a good trick when you are encouraging young children to eat vegetables and it often works. Last but not least, check the labelling on tinned tomatoes, pasata and tomato purée. High fructose corn syrup is sometimes added.

## Aubergine Melanzane

*One of the delights of Italian cooking that has found its way around the world. Melanzane benefits from being cooked and then reheated as this allows the flavours develop. It freezes very well. Serve it with a simple green salad or some green vegetables.*

SERVES 4
1½ kg/3lbs Aubergine
2 tbsp olive oil ( or the oil from the tin of anchovies)
500ml/18fl oz Passata (sieved tomato)
3 tbsp Tomato purée
2 tsp vegetable stock powder
250g/8oz) Mozzarella or Feta
2 - 3 cloves of garlic - crushed
Finely grated parmesan
Large handful of basil leaves
2 tbsp chopped black olives and/or capers
80g Tin anchovy fillets in olive oil

Pre heat the oven to 180°C/ 350°F/Gas 4

1 Slice the aubergines about 5mm/¼in thick.. Put them into a microwave bowl, cover and microwave on full power for about 5 minutes until they are soft.

2 Heat the Passata, stir in the tomato concentrate, the bouillon powder, the crushed garlic and the oil. Leave to simmer on a low heat for about 10 minutes.

3 Grease a wide shallow ovenproof dish or tin. Put a layer of the cooked aubergine over the base, then add some tomato sauce, some torn basil leaves, olives or capers, some of the cheese and a scatter of parmesan.. Add another layer of aubergine, tomato sauce, basil, cheese and olives and finish with a layer of tomato.

4 Tear up the anchovy fillets and scatter them over the top. Bake for 45 minutes.

## Spinach & Red Pepper Moussaka

*This is a cross between a spinach pie and a Moussaka. Traditionally a spinach pie is cooked in a case of filo pastry and a moussaka is made with a meat stew that is cooked between layers of aubergine. Like most aubergine dishes this moussaka freezes well so you can freeze any leftovers or make it in advance especially for the freezer. If you do freeze it you do not need to complete the final baking process. You can use fresh peppers that you roast yourself or you can use ready roasted peppers that are sold in jars and cans.*

SERVES 4

600g/1lb 5oz aubergine plus olive oil for brushing
400g /14 oz cooked spinach or Swiss chard
2 tbsp pine nuts lightly toasted
200g /7 oz feta crumbled
6 spring onions finely sliced
3 large red peppers OR a jar of roasted red peppers

For the béchamel sauce
40g / 1½oz plain flour
500ml / 18 fl oz milk
60g / 2oz grated parmesan
1 egg beaten
Grated nutmeg and ground black pepper.

Preheat the oven to 180°C/ 350°F/Gas 4 and Grease a large dish, about 5cm/2 inches deep.

1. Slice the aubergines into rounds 1cm /½ inch thick. Line two baking trays with foil and brush them with oil. Put the sliced aubergines onto the trays and lightly brush them with oil. Bake them at 180°C for 15 minutes. The aubergine should be soft but not brown. Put the cooked aubergine to one side
2. If you are using fresh red peppers, turn the oven up to 200°C/ 400°F/Gas 5. Cut the red peppers in quarters and roast them for 30 minutes until the skin is beginning to blister and look charred. Put them into a dish, cover them with cling film and leave them to cool a little. Peel the skins off of the peppers and tear them into strips.

Reserve any oil that has come out of them.

3. Make the béchamel sauce. Melt the butter on a gentle heat and stir in the flour. Cook gently for a couple of minutes. You do not want the flour to take on any colour.
4. Using a whisk, slowly add the milk and keep whisking. Most recipes tell you to warm the milk when making a sauce to prevent lumps forming. If you use a whisk there is no need to warm the milk. When all the milk is added stir in the grated parmesan and cook gently for 5 minutes, stirring occasionally. Turn off the heat.
5. Squeeze the spinach or chard to make sure it is dry and mix it with the toasted pine nuts, chopped spring onions and the crumbled feta.
6. Pour about a quarter of the béchamel sauce over the bottom of the dish and place a layer of the cooked aubergine on top. Add the spinach mixture and on top of this pour another quarter of the béchamel sauce.
7. Put in another layer of cooked aubergine and then the red peppers. Top the peppers with the remaining aubergine.
8. Beat the egg and mix it with the remaining béchamel sauce and pour this over the top layer of aubergine. Bake for 45 minutes. Serve with a green salad or some green vegetables.

## Pumpkin, Tomato & Chestnut Bake

*You can use pumpkin, butternut squash or sweet potatoes to make this.*

SERVES 4

1½ Kg/3lb 6 oz small pumpkin or butternut squash
1 tsp oregano
1 tsp chilli flakes
1 tbsp olive oil
200g/7oz cherry tomatoes
2 balls mozzarella cheese cut into slices
Small handful of basil leaves
12 cooked chestnuts cut into quarters
2 tbsp balsamic vinegar
60g/2¼oz packet baby spinach leaves

Pre heat the oven to 200°C/ 400°F/Gas 5

1. Peel the pumpkin or butternut squash, remove the seeds and chop it into large chunks. Put it into a bowl and add the olive oil, oregano and chilli flakes and season to taste.
2. Put the pumpkin or butter squash onto a roasting tray lined with non stick foil and bake for 20 minutes. Turn it over half way through.
3. Add the cherry tomatoes and the chestnuts and turn them over with the pumpkin or squash. Cook for 10 minutes.
4. Stir in the mozzarella and basil leaves and drizzle over the balsamic vinegar before serving on a bed of baby spinach leaves

## Beans In Red Mole Sauce

*This is a taste of Mexico at its best and yes, it really does contain cocoa. As the sauce freezes well it is worth making a batch for the freezer. If you do decide to freeze it leave out the garlic as this can give rise to a slightly musty flavour.*

*You can add any type of bean or vegetable to the sauce and it also works well with firm tofu or tempeh and the micro protein Quorn, either as a 'Quorn Mince' or as 'Quorn chunks'.*

---

SERVES 6

For the sauce
2 tbsp olive oil
1 large red onion finely chopped
3 cloves garlic crushed
3 tbsp cocoa powder
1 tsp chilli powder
2 tsp ground cumin
1 tsp smoked paprika
1 tbsp sweet paprika
½ tsp salt
1 tbsp dried oregano
2 x 400g/14oz cans chopped tomatoes
2 red peppers finely sliced or diced
400g/14 oz can red or black beans
400g/14 oz black eyed beans

Avocado Salsa:
4 tbsp finely chopped fresh coriander
1 large avocado
Juice of half a lemon or a whole lime
1 tbsp finely chopped red onion

Natural unsweetened Greek style yoghurt to serve

---

1 Reserve a small hand full of the red peppers for a garnish. Heat the olive oil in a large saucepan. Add the onion, garlic and the rest of the red peppers and sauté over a medium heat for 5 to 10 minutes. Do not let the onion or garlic brown.
2 In a small bowl mix together the cocoa powder, chilli, cumin, both types of paprika, salt and oregano. Add this to the onion and pepper mixture, stir well and cook, stirring all the time, for a minute or two to bring out the flavour of the spices.
3 Add the canned tomatoes. Give everything a good stir, bring to the

boil, turn down the heat and simmer gently for 10 minutes. Pre heat the oven to 160°C/ 325°F/Gas 3

4 Drain and rinse the beans and add them to the sauce. Bring everything back to the boil, then turn off the heat and transfer the beans and sauce to an oven proof dish or casserole. Cook for 30 – 40 minutes while you prepare the salsa.

5 Cut the avocado in half. Remove the stone using a small spoon, then peel and chop it into small pieces. Stir in the lemon juice and add the finely chopped red onion and the chopped coriander.

Serve the beans garnished with the reserved red peppers and with the natural yoghurt and the avocado salsa in separate bowls.

## Chinese Leaf, Pepper & Sweetcorn Salad

*Chinese leaf is a valuable store cupboard ingredient as it is available all the year round and it keeps well. This is a bright, colourful salad that will keep for 2 days in a covered container in the fridge. Serve it on its own or with a dressing of your choice.*

SERVES 4 - 6

1 large sweet Ramiro pepper
325g/11 ½oz can sweetcorn kernels
4 spring onions finely sliced
½ Chinese Leaf Cabbage
2 punnets of mustard cress

1 Remove the seeds from the red pepper and cut it into thin rings. Finely shred the Chinese Leaf.

2 Rinse and drain the sweetcorn kernels, put them into a large bowl and mix them with the mustard cress.

3 Stir in the red pepper and Chinese Leaf and the spring onions.

## Tomato & Lentil Soup

*This is a basic soup that you can easily transform into something completely different by simply changing the herbs and spices you use.*

SERVES 4

400g/14oz tin chopped tomatoes
3 tbsp tomato purée
1 large red onion roughly chopped
1 stick celery roughly chopped
1 large carrot roughly chopped
100g/3½oz red lentils
1 tbsp olive oil
1tsp Sambol Oelek or ½ tsp chilli powder (optional)
700ml/25 fl oz/1¼pt vegetable stock
3 cloves of garlic roughly chopped
4 tbsp natural unsweetened Greek style yoghurt
handful of torn basil leaves

1. Wash and pick over the red lentils and make sure that there is no grit in them. Leave them to drain while you prepare the vegetables.
2. Heat the olive oil and lightly sauté the onion, garlic, celery and carrot for 3 or 4 minutes. Don't let them brown. Add the tin of chopped tomatoes, the tomato purée, the Sambol Oelek and chilli.
3. Add the vegetable stock and the lentils. Give everything a good stir, bring it to the boil, cover and simmer for 30 - 40 minutes until the lentils are tender.
4. Using a hand blender blend the soup until it is smooth. Stir in the yoghurt and the torn basil leaves.

*Variation:*

You can give this soup a Middle Eastern flavour by omitting the yoghurt and basil and adding 1 tsp ground cumin, 1 tsp dried dill and ½ tsp ground cardamom seeds when you add the tin of tomatoes.

## English Onion Soup

*This soup scores high on the anti inflammation scale and it is also a really simple soup to make. The dry vermouth and grated raw onion added at the end give it an extra special twist. If you have some truffle oil just a small amount sprinkled on when the soup is served tastes amazing. The soup freezes well and can be stored in the fridge for up to 2 days.*

---

SERVES 4

700g/1 lb 9 oz onions peeled and thinly sliced
2 tbsp grated onion
400g/14oz potatoes peeled and sliced
3 tbsp olive oil
1.7Lt/3pt vegetable stock
4 tbsp dry vermouth (optional)
4 tbsp fromage frais or natural unsweetened yoghurt
¼ tsp grated nutmeg
salt and pepper to taste

4 tbsp grated parmesan to serve OR some truffle oil

---

1. Heat the olive oil in a large saucepan and add the sliced onions and
2. the potato. Sauté them for 5 minutes and then add the stock. Bring to the boil, cover, reduce the heat and simmer them for 20 minutes until the potatoes and onions are tender.
3. Use a hand blender to blend the soup until it is smooth. Add the dry vermouth if you are using it and season to taste with the grated nutmeg, salt and black pepper.
4. When you are ready to serve the soup stir in the grated onion and fromage frais. Serve the grated Parmesan in a separate bowl.

## Mexican Bean Burgers & Guacamole

*These are quick and easy to make and as they freeze well it is worth making a large batch for the freezer. Serve the burgers with a green salad and guacamole.*

SERVES

200g/7oz finely chopped red onion
200g/7oz red cabbage finely sliced
2 x 400g/14 oz cans red kidney beans, drained and rinsed
175g/6oz firm tofu
2 tbsp olive oil
2 tsp ground cumin
2 tsp smoked paprika
2 tbsp sweet paprika
1 tsp chilli powder
4 tbsp chopped coriander
150g/5½oz cooked millet
Fine polenta or toasted oatmeal coating

1. Heat the oil in a saucepan and fry the red onion and the red cabbage for a few minutes. Keep stirring to prevent the cabbage from sticking. Turn down the heat to low and add the ground cumin, the smoked paprika, the sweet paprika and the chilli power. Give everything a quick stir and then add about 3 tbsp water. Cover the pan and cook for 20 minutes. Stir it occasionally to make sure it is not sticking. Leave the onion and cabbage to cool for about half an hour.
2. Put the tofu with half of the red beans and half of the onion and cabbage mixture into a bowl and blitz them with a hand blender until you have a slightly chunky paste.
3. Add the rest of the red beans, the rest of the onion and cabbage mixture and the chopped coriander. Blend lightly. You want to have the burgers blended enough for everything to stick together. You want some whole beans and pieces of cabbage. You don't want to turn it into a mush. Stir in the cooked millet and leave the mixture to cool for an hour or two before moving on to the next stage.
4. Put some fine polenta or toasted oatmeal coating onto a plate. Flour your hands with it, take a large heaped tablespoon of the mixture and form it into a burger shapes about 7cm/3in in diameter. Put the

burgers onto a tray lined with cling film or non stick foil and put them into the fridge until you cook them. At this stage you can also freeze them.

5 To cook the burgers, oil a large non stick pan and fry them for 5 minutes on each side until a crust forms. Alternatively, lightly brush them with oil, put them onto a non stick baking tray and bake them at 200°C/ 400°F/Gas 5 for 15 to 20 minutes.

## Toasted Oatmeal Coating

*This is a useful mixture of oatmeal, spices and seeds that can be used as a crunchy topping for bakes an gratins and as a coating for burgers.*

SERVES 4
200g/7oz flaked oatmeal
3 tbsp olive oil
3 tbsp water
A handful of sunflower seeds
½ tsp ground turmeric
1 tsp garlic granules
1 tbsp dried oregano
1 tsp chilli flakes

Pre heat the oven to 160°C/ 325°F/Gas 3

Grease a 20cm/8 in square baking tin and line the base with baking parchment or non stick foil.

1. Mix the flaked oats and sunflower seeds with the turmeric, garlic granules, chilli flakes and oregano.
2. Put the water and olive oil into a saucepan and bring it to the boil.
3. Add the oil and water for the flaked oats. Mix well and press the mixture into the prepared tin. Bake for 30 minutes until the oats are golden brown.
4. Leave the oats to cool completely, then use a rolling pin to break the oats down into large crumbs. Store in an airtight tin or freeze.

## Guacamole

*They say that an authentic Guacamole contains only avocado, fresh coriander, tomato and fresh chillies. If you add anything else to it it becomes an avocado dip.*

*You can use this recipe as a dip by adding some natural unsweetened yoghurt and serve it with raw vegetables and pieces of Socca and you can use it as a sauce with cold fish and bean dishes and with Mexican burgers. When serving it with beans it works really well with red beans.*

*Use really ripe avocados for the best results. You can alter the proportions of the various ingredients to suit your taste.*

---

SERVES

2 to 3 fresh chillies finely chopped
OR 2 tsp Sambol Oelek
2 medium tomatoes finely chopped
1 tbsp finely chopped onion
1 clove garlic crushed
2 tbsp chopped fresh coriander
2 large or 3 medium ripe avocados
Lemon or lime juice to taste

---

1 Peel and mash the avocado and mix it with the other ingredients.

2 Add 1 or 2 tablespoons of lemon juice and mix well. Leave the stone in the guacamole until you are ready to eat it as for some reason this slows down the oxidation process.

3 Do not refrigerate. If you do the guacamole will go brown.

## Fish:- especially oily cold water fish

### Why?

Fish contain large amounts of fatty acids and these, especially Omega-3 essential fatty acids, have powerful anti-inflammatory properties. Fish is also an excellent sources of protein and other vital nutrients, including antioxidants. Yes, like all animal products fish contains iron but in much smaller amounts than red meat. The health giving benefits of the Omega-3 essential fatty acids far outweigh any disadvantages of the iron. Cold water oily fish like salmon, sardines, herring, mackerel, trout, and halibut are all excellent sources of Omega-3 but all fish, including shellfish and seafood are a good choice as part of a gout diet, even white fish. Forget about the dire warnings about purines. Prawns, mussels and oysters are back on the menu.

### How?

Substitute fish for meat in your diet and try to eat it four times a week. There is very good evidence that a diet high in fish and fish oils is of great benefit if you suffer from gout. Now, unless you live near the coast or have access to a good fishmonger, fresh fish is not so easy to obtain. Trout and salmon can usually be found but other than this you will probably have to buy frozen fish. Just remember to thaw it slowly and then wash and dry it thoroughly in order to remove any oils that have oxidised. Unfortunately oily fish like sardines, herring and mackerel do not freeze well so you may have to resort to tins. Just make sure the fish is tinned in water or olive oil and not sunflower oil. One way the northern Europeans preserve their oily fish, especially herring, is to pickle it. Bismark herrings and roll mops are usually sold in jars and as they require no cooking they are quick and easy to prepare. Despite the fact that they are salted and then preserved in vinegar that is sometimes sweetened this type of fish is a very valuable source of healthy oils.

The only downside to fish is that levels of mercury can sometimes be high, so should you be worried about mercury in fish?

Because it is exposed to environmental pollution all fish and shellfish contain mercury. Some types of fish contain only trace amounts while others contain much more.

Mercury is a problem because too much can deactivate some important enzymes in our bodies that are dependent on selenium. However, in addition to mercury, fish and seafood contains selenium and while we are given dire warnings about the dangers of mercury, what we are not told is that provided the fish we eat contains more selenium than mercury there is no danger. With the exception of pilot whale, shark, tilefish, swordfish and king mackerel, fish contains more selenium than mercury, so cod, salmon, trout, haddock, herring and sardines are perfectly safe to eat. It is interesting to note that according to the US National Fisheries Institute there has never been a confirmed case of mercury poisoning in the United States that was caused by eating fish or seafood.

Most of the salmon and trout we eat today is farmed. As well as ethical issues about health, welfare and the food the farmed fish are fed on, farmed fish contains less Omega-3 oils and more Omega-6 oils than wild fish. But when you compare the 1,100mg of Omega-3 a 125 gram portion of oily fish contains to the 35mg found in the same amount of lean grass fed beef, it is clear to see how important fish is in a healthy diet. We are all getting mixed messages about eating fish, but irrespective of whether it is wild or farmed eating fish leads to a massive improvement in our intake of Omega 3 fatty acids, something that is in very short supply in our modern Western diet. At the end of the day, in terms of overall nutritional value, you need to look at the big picture and use this to make your decisions.

**Tip:**

Fish cooks very quickly so try not to overcook it. With oily fish the oils oxidise quite easily and its nutritional value reduces the longer it is cooked. Steaming, poaching, baking or lightly sautéed is a much better option than frying or grilling. When you are cooking fish in a pan cover the pan for half of the cooking time. The trapped moisture will steam the fish and as a bonus you can produce a fine sauce from the fluid in the pan.

## Herring With Beetroot & Horseradish

*This is one of those almost instant meals especially if you have some quinoa already cooked in the freezer. You can use Bismark Herrings or Roll mops to make this recipe. These are ready to eat and usually sold in jars or plastic tubs. The herrings need to be stored in the fridge but as they have a fairly long shelf life they are a useful store cupboard ingredient. All you need to do is drain them before using them in the recipe.*

SERVES 4

Large jar 500g/1lb 2oz of Bismarck Herring or Roll mops
100g/3½oz quinoa
230ml/8 fl oz water
500g/1lb 2oz packet of cooked beetroot
Half a medium red onion finely chopped
1 telegraph cucumber
3 – 4 heaped tsp grated horseradish
Juice of a lemon
1 tbsp olive oil (optional)
50g/1¾oz packet baby salad leaves, baby spinach or rocket

To Serve
4 tbsp fromage frais
1 tbsp finely chopped fresh dill
1 tbsp finely chopped capers

1 Quinoa is not the easiest of grains to cook as it needs long, very slow cooking. The easiest way to cook it is by using the absorption method. 100G/3½ oz of quinoa will need approximately 230ml/8 fl oz of water.
2 Wash the quinoa and drain it. Put it into a saucepan, bring it to the boil, cover and reduce to a very, very low heat. Leave it to cook for 25 – 30 minutes. When it has finished cooking leave it to stand for at least a quarter of an hour before taking the lid off. Alternatively cook the Quinoa in the microwave following the instructions in the Grains and Rice section.
3 Leave the Quinoa to cool while you prepare the rest of the ingredients.

4 Mix the horseradish with the lemon juice and if you are using it, the olive oil in a jam jar. Put on the lid and give it a good shake.

5 Peel the cucumber, cut it in half lengthways and remove the seeds. Chop it into small 5mm/¼ in dice.

6 Rinse and dry the beetroot and cut it into small 5mm/¼ in dice. Stir the chopped red onion, cucumber, horseradish and lemon juice into the Quinoa.

7 Cut the Herrings into bite size pieces and either place them on top or mix them with the beetroot and quinoa. You can keep this salad in the fridge for up to 24 hours.

8 Mix the fromage frais with the chopped dill and capers and serve it in a separate bowl. Serve the Quinoa and herrings on a bed of salad leaves or rocket.

## Cullen Skink

*Cullen Skink is a traditional Scottish fish stew with a history that goes back hundreds of years. You do not need to stick rigidly to the recipe as you can make the soup from just about any fish or shellfish that you have available. However, the one thing you do need to include is some smoked fish, preferably fish that has been naturally smoked and not dyed.*

SERVES 4

1 large leek
1 medium onion
1 stick of celery very finely sliced
2 tbsp butter
2 tbsp plain flour
600ml/20fl oz (1pt) milk
300ml/10 fl oz (½pt) water
2 large potatoes peeled and cut into small cubes
450g/1lb un-dyed smoked haddock with skin and bones removed
115g/4oz small courgette cut into small dice
225g/8oz white fish with skin and bones removed
225g/8oz salmon with skin and bones removed
16 frozen mussels, shells removed

1. Slice the leek and onion thinly. Cut the fish into small 1cm/½in dice. Melt the butter in a large saucepan and fry the leek, onion and celery over a medium heat for about 5 minutes.
2. Still with the pan on a medium heat, stir in the flour and cook it for 2 minutes stirring it occasionally, Be careful not to let it brown. Add the milk and water and stir until the liquid comes to the boil and thickens. If you turn the heat too high the sauce at the bottom of the saucepan will stick and burn.
3. Add the potatoes and bring the soup back to the boil. Reduce the heat to very low and simmer for 15 minutes or until the potatoes are tender.
4. Increase the heat a little and add the courgettes, the fish and the mussels and bring the soup to the boil. Turn the heat back to low and simmer for 5 – 7 minutes. Season with black pepper and garnish with some finely chopped chives or chopped dill before serving.

## Red Peppers Stuffed with Mackerel

*Many vegetables lend themselves to being stuffed and the ingredients you use for the stuffing can be quite versatile. This a simple recipe that can be prepared very quickly. You can use any type of fresh or canned fish. The fish used in this recipe is a 'No Drain' can of mackerel fillets that have no added oil. This type of fish is a useful store cupboard ingredient.*

SERVES 2

2 large red bell peppers
1 large potato weighing about 350g/12oz
110g/4oz tin 'no drain' mackerel fillets
1tsp chilli paste or Sambol Oelek
1 heaped tsp dried dill
2 - 3 spring onions finely sliced
50g/1¾oz prawns (optional)
1 tbsp Thai fish sauce

Pre heat the oven to 180°C/ 350°F/Gas 4

1 Prick the potato and cook it in a microwave on full power for 5 minutes. Turn it over and cook for another 3 -4 minutes until it is just soft. As soon as the potato is cool enough to handle peel off the skin and either mash it or put it through a potato ricer.

2 Cut the peppers in half lengthways through the stem. Remove the seeds and any white pith.

3 Put the peppers cut side up into a lightly greased oven proof pan. You may need to trim the round side a little so that they sit flat. If you end up with a hole put the piece you trimmed off back inside to fill the gap.

4 Break the mackerel fillets into smallish chunks and mix them with the prawns, dill, spring onions, Sambol Oelek and Thai fish sauce into the mashed potato. Divide the mixture between the halved peppers and press it down well.

5 Bake the peppers uncovered for 20 - 25 minutes or until they feel soft when tested with a sharp knife.

## Fish Baked in Tomato & Cardamom Sauce

*This recipe originates from the Middle East. It is a basic tomato sauce that can be used with any type of white fish or shellfish, tilapia works well. If you leave out the garlic you can make a large batch of the sauce and store it in the freezer. Adjust the amount of chilli or Sambol Oelek you use to suit your taste.*

SERVES 4

400g/14oz can chopped tomatoes
3 tbsp tomato purée
1 medium white or red onion chopped
1 tbsp olive oil
3 cloves garlic crushed
1 chopped chilli or 1 tsp Sambol Oelek
4 tbsp chopped fresh dill OR 2 tsp dried dill
2 tsp ground cumin
1 tsp ground cardamom
Ground black pepper to taste
4x fillets white fish weighing about 150g/5½oz each
Juice 1 lemon (optional)

Pre heat the oven to 180°C/ 350°F/Gas 4

1 Heat the olive oil in a saucepan or frying pan. Add the onion and garlic sauté for 3 – 4 minutes.

2 Add the chilli or Sambol Oelek, the cardamom, the cumin and the dill, give it a good stir and then add the tinned tomatoes and the tomato purée. Leave the sauce to cook gently over a low heat while you prepare the fish.

3 Wash and dry the fish and put it into a greased baking dish that is large enough to lay the fish in a single layer. Pour over the tomato sauce. Cover with foil and bake in the middle of the oven for 20 - 25 minutes depending on the thickness of the fish. The fish should be set and translucent.

## Niçoise Salad

*A classic way of serving fresh, frozen or tinned tuna and transforming a small amount of fish into a substantial meal. You can vary both the amount and type of vegetables you use depending on what you have available. If you use frozen tuna try to buy yellow fin tuna steaks that are vacuum packed in individual bags. These are less oxidised and have a much better flavour than the ordinary 'dark' tuna. Don't be put off by the long list of ingredients. This is a very easy recipe to make.*

SERVES 4

350g/12oz cherry tomatoes cut in half
110g/4 oz rocket or baby salad leaves
½ telegraph cucumber
175g/6oz fine French beans
450g/1lb cooked small new potatoes OR 400g/14oz can cannellini beans drained and rinsed
8 spring onions sliced
3 - 4 large free range eggs that have been hard boiled
1 tbsp finely chopped flat leaf parsley
20 salted black olives with their stones removed
400g/14oz tin 'no drain' tuna steak OR 4 x small pieces of frozen tuna

For the dressing:
Cooking fluid from the tuna
½ clove garlic crushed
1 tbsp seeded mustard
2 tbsp finely grated parmesan
1 tbsp lemon juice
1 heaped tsp anchovy paste

1 If you are using frozen tuna defrost it slowly at room temperature and then wash and dry it in kitchen paper. Cut each tuna steak in half horizontally into thin pieces.
2 Mix 1 tbsp olive oil with 2 tbsp lemon juice and put it into a saucepan. Bring it to a gentle simmer and then add the pieces of tuna. Bring it back to simmering point, cover and cook for 3 minutes. Turn the slices of tune over and cook them for another 2 minutes. Take if off the heat and leave the tuna to cool while you prepare the salad.

3 Put the French beans into a pan of boiling water. Bring them to the boil and cook them for 3 minutes. Drain them, refresh them in cold water, drain them again and put them to one side.
4 Cut the cucumber in half lengthways and remove the seeds. Cut each half of the cucumber into thin crescent shaped slices.
5 Peel the hard boiled eggs and cut them into quarters.
6 Slice the cooked new potatoes into thin slices.
7 Put the French beans, tomatoes, sliced cucumber, potatoes, olives and spring onions into a bowl and mix well.
8 To make the dressing drain the cooking liquid from the tuna into a jar and mix it with the anchovy paste, crushed garlic, seeded mustard, parmesan and lemon juice. Give it a really good shake to combine the ingredients.
9 When you are ready to serve the salad mix the rocket with the other ingredients and arrange it on a serving plate. Put the pieces of tuna on top and arrange the hard boiled eggs around the edge. Sprinkle on the chopped parsley, Serve the dressing in a separate bowl.

## Tuna & Borlotti Bean Salad

*This is a famous dish from Tuscany that is one of those 'instant' out of the store cupboard meals. You will need good quality tuna, preferably a 'no drain' brand as you do not want the salad swimming in brine or oil.*

SERVES 2 - 4

400g/14oz borlotti or cannellini beans drained and rinsed
120g/4¼ oz can 'no drain' tuna steak in spring water
3 spring onions cut into match stick size slices
Salt and pepper to taste
2 tbsp lemon juice
2 tbsp olive oil
1 tbsp finely chopped parsley or chervil.
50g/1¾oz cooked fine French Beans (optional)
30g/1oz baby spinach leaves

1 Put the olive oil and lemon juice together in a jar and give it a good shake.

2 Mix the borlotti beans, spring onions and, if you using them, the French Beans together in a bowl and stir in the dressing.

3 Break the tuna into small pieces and arrange them on top of the beans. Scatter the parsley or chervil on top and serve on a bed of baby spinach leaves.

## Creole Tuna Salad

*This tuna salad is far removed from the more usual 'tuna, sweetcorn and mayonnaise' salad. It is one of those salads that you can make from more or less any ingredients that you have available and it is most definitely more salad than fish. As with the borlotti bean and tuna salad you need good quality 'no drain' tuna steak.*

SERVES 2 – 4

1 large carrot coarsely grated
1 red pepper finely chopped
½ small red onion finely chopped
1 small green under ripe mango
1 green chilli finely chopped OR
1 tsp Sambol Oelek or chilli paste
50g/1¾oz finely shredded cabbage or Chinese leaf
120g/4¼ oz can 'no drain' tuna steak in spring water
Finely grated zest and juice of a lime
2 tbsp chopped coriander or what ever herbs you have available
2 tbsp lightly toasted pumpkin and sunflower seeds

1 Remove the stone from the mango. Peel it and cut it into 1cm/½ in chunks. Put it into a large bowl and stir in the lime zest, lime juice and chopped chilli.
2 Add the grated carrot, red pepper, chopped onion and shredded cabbage.
3 Break up the tuna on a plate and stir it in. Garnish with the chopped herbs and toasted seeds.

Serve with green or red Tabasco or hot pepper sauce.

## Nuts and Seeds

### Why?

Nuts and seeds are complex foods that contain many different nutrients, some of which are known to reduce chronic and systemic inflammation and inflammatory markers. They are loaded with healthy Omega-3 and Omega-6 essential fatty acids that are in a 'natural' ratio and they bring with them their own supply of antioxidants and vitamins that stop the oil oxidising. Walnuts, almonds, hazelnuts, pumpkin seeds, sesame seeds, flax seeds, in fact all nuts and seeds are good and they are great for snacking on.

Isn't Omega-6 one of the not so good oils? Well nuts and seeds are not just tiny packets of Omega-6. They are a long way from the heat processed polyunsaturated vegetable oils. As nuts and seeds are something a tree or plant grows from they are a pretty complete source of nutrition; fats, carbohydrates, and protein plus vitamins like vitamin E, minerals and antioxidants that protect the fats from becoming oxidised. When we strip the oil from the seed it doesn't have any of these things to protect it and this is when the trouble starts. A hand full of nuts bares no resemblance to a spoonful of hot pressed vegetable oil.

### How?

Only buy natural uncooked nuts and seeds. Commercially roasted nuts and seeds usually contain a lot of additives and you have no control over how long they have been roasted for or the temperature they have been roasted at. Polyunsaturated vegetable oils are also often added as part of the roasting process. You can soak seeds overnight to make them plump and succulent or roast them lightly. If you cook them too much the oils in them oxidise and the antioxidants they contain are reduced.

Use them as a sprinkle on salads and vegetables. Try adding them to cooked bulgar wheat and quinoa. Tahini, a paste made from lightly toasted sesame seeds is widely used in Mediterranean and North African cooking. It can be added to vegetables and ground or puréed beans and it can be used as a dressing for warm and cold salads.

## Onion & Walnut Muffins

*Onions in a muffin? Well yes, and interestingly they do not have a strong onion taste. These savoury muffins are great for breakfast and they also go really well with soup. You can use walnuts or pecan nuts to make them. The muffins taste good and the onions and nuts make them a special anti-inflammatory treat. If you are avoiding wheat use a mixture of fine oatmeal and buckwheat instead of the spelt. These muffins freeze well so make twice the quantity and put some into the freezer.*

---

Makes 8 large muffins or 12 small ones

125g/4½oz white onion roughly chopped
4 tbsp olive oil
1 large free range egg
1 tsp cayenne pepper
1 tsp garlic granules
1 tsp baking powder
150g/5½oz finely chopped pecan nuts or walnuts
175g/6oz wholegrain spelt

---

Pre heat the oven to 220°C/ 450°F/Gas 6 and grease your muffin tins.

1 Put the walnuts into a blender or food processor and process until they are finely chopped.

2 Put the ground walnuts into a bowl with the spelt and baking powder and mix well.

3 Put the chopped onion with the olive oil, egg, cayenne pepper and garlic granules into a food processor or blender and whiz until you have a smooth purée.

4 Add the onion and egg purée to the walnut and spelt and mix thoroughly. Spoon into muffin tins and bake for 5 minutes then turn the oven down to 200°C/ 400°F/Gas 5 and cook for another 15 minutes.

## Goats Cheese & Walnut Salad

*A simple salad that takes only minutes to prepare. Goats cheese, walnuts or pecan nuts and red beans go together really well. If you don't like goats cheese use Camembert or Brie instead.*

SERVES 4

250g/9oz Chevre log cut into16 pieces
16 slices from a small baguette cut ½ cm/¼ in thick
70g/2½oz packet of mixed baby salad leaves
400g/14 oz can red beans drained and rinsed
85g/3oz walnuts or pecan nuts roughly chopped
Small bunch chives cut into 2cm/1 in pieces

For the dressing:
1 tbsp walnut oil
1 tbsp lemon juice
½ tsp chilli paste or Sambol Oelek

1 Set the grill onto high and toast the slices of baguette on one side.

2 Put the salad leaves into a large bowl with the red beans and the walnuts. Mix the walnut oil, chilli and lemon juice together and mix it into the salad and beans. Divide the salad between 4 plates.

3 Put the slices of Chevre onto the un-toasted side of the baguette and grill it until it turns a light golden brown. Keep an eye on it as it burns very easily.

4 Arrange 4 pieces of the grilled Chevre log on top of the salad and serve immediately.

## Red Cabbage, Bean & Walnut Salad

*This is a variation on a traditional red bean and walnut salad from the Caucuses. While in no way authentic, the pickled walnuts give this version of the salad its characteristic flavour. If you are unable to obtain pickled walnuts increase the amount of walnuts and use some Worcestershire Sauce instead of the pickled walnut vinegar. Serve the salad as an appetiser or as part of a main meal. It works particularly well with savoury cheesecakes.*

SERVES 4

½ small red cabbage very finely shredded
1 medium red onion finely sliced
400g/14oz can red beans drained and rinsed
50g/1¾oz finely chopped walnuts
1 pickled walnut finely chopped
2 tbsp walnut oil
2 tbsp pickled walnut vinegar
1 tsp chilli paste or Sambol Oelek
1 clove garlic crushed (optional)
Juice and finely grated zest of a lime
2 tbsp finely chopped coriander OR 1 tbsp ready made coriander pesto

1 Mix together the walnuts, pickled walnuts, vinegar, walnut oil, chilli, lime juice, grated lime zest, crushed garlic and coriander.

2 Mix together the cabbage, red onion and beans, stir in the dressing, cover and chill. The salad will keep for 2 days in a covered container in the fridge.

## Brazil Nut & Vegetable Korma

*A creamy lightly spiced curry. Like most spiced dishes it benefits from being made in advance so that the flavours can develop.*

SERVES 4

50g/1¾oz creamed coconut
2 tbsp olive oil
2 medium onions chopped
2 fresh red or green chillies or
2 tsp chilli paste
1 tsp ground cumin
1 tsp ground turmeric
1 tsp ground coriander
1 clove crushed garlic
125g/4 oz ground Brazil nuts or cashew nuts
1 small cauliflower broken into florets
250g/8 oz courgettes sliced
125g/4 oz sugar snaps
125g/4 oz cooked peas
4 tbsp fresh chopped coriander

1. Roughly chop the coconut and dissolve it in 450ml/16fl oz of boiling water. Heat the olive oil and fry the onion for 5 minutes, stirring occasionally. Add the chillies, garlic and spices. Stir well and cook for 2 minutes over a medium heat.
2. Stir the ground Brazil nuts into the coconut water and then add this to the onion and spices. Bring it to simmering point, cover and turn the heat to low. You can prepare the recipe to this stage and store it overnight in the fridge.
3. Put some water into a saucepan and bring it to the boil. Add the cauliflower and cook for 3 minutes. Stir in the sugar snaps, bring back to the boil, cover and turn off the heat.
4. While the cauliflower is cooking steam the courgettes in a microwave for 3 minutes.
5. Drain the cauliflower and sugar snaps and add them with the courgettes and cooked peas to the nut, spice and onion mixture. Serve garnished with chopped coriander.

## Celery & Almond Roast

*You can use silken tofu or a low fat cheese like Quark or Ricotta. The roast can be eaten hot or cold. It does not freeze but it will keep in the fridge for 2 to 3 days.*

SERVES 4 – 6

350g/12oz silken tofu
500g/1lb 2oz celery finely sliced
100g/3½oz flaked oats
4 tbsp finely grated parmesan
200g/7oz toasted flaked almonds
2 tbsp chopped parsley
½tsp ground turmeric
3 free range eggs
finely grated zest of a lemon
juice of a lemon

Heat the oven to 180°C/ 350°F/Gas 4

1. Put the finely sliced celery into a microwave bowl, cover and cook on full power for 5 minutes. Give it a stir, put the cover back on and cook for another 5 minutes. Leave it to cool slightly.
2. Put the flaked almonds onto a baking tray and bake them for 6 minutes. Just long enough for them to take on some colour.
3. Put the silken tofu into a large bowl, add the eggs, turmeric and lemon zest and give everything a whiz with a hand blender until the tofu is thoroughly amalgamated with the eggs.
4. Stir in the grated parmesan, the flaked oats, parsley, celery, toasted almonds and lemon juice.
5. Grease a 1½Kg/3lb 6oz loaf tin, spoon in the mixture and press it down. Cover with foil and bake for 30 minutes at 180°C/ 350°F/Gas 4.
6. Turn the oven down to 160°C/ 325°F/Gas 3, take off the foil and cook for another 30 minutes. Leave the roast to stand for 10 – 15 minutes before turning it out of the tin.

## Brazil Nut & Oatmeal Tiffin

*Quick and easy to make this recipe uses lightly toasted Brazil nuts and fine oatmeal instead of digestive biscuits,*

---

MAKES 16

175g/6oz flaked oats
125g/4½oz Brazil nuts
85g/3oz butter
4 heaped tbsp raisins soaked for ½ hour in hot water
3 tbsp cocoa powder
3 heaped tbsp dark unrefined sugar
4 tbsp water
1 tsp vanilla extract
75g/2¾ oz 70% or 85% chocolate

---

You will need a 20cm/8 in square tin to make this. Pre heat the oven to 180°C/ 350°F/Gas 4.

1. Put the flaked oats and Brazil nuts into a food processor or blender and process until they form a smooth fairly fine powder. Put them onto a baking tray and bake them for 5 minutes. Take them out of the oven and give them a good stir. Put them back into the oven and cook for another 5 minutes. They should look lightly toasted. Put them to one side while you prepare the rest of the ingredients.
2. Put the butter, water, cocoa powder and sugar into a medium size saucepan and gently heat it until the butter is melted. Keep stirring it over a low heat and cook it for 3 – 4 minutes. This will take the raw taste out of the cocoa.
3. Stir in the vanilla extract and raisins, then add the baked oatmeal and Brazil nuts. Mix thoroughly. The mixture will be quite stiff. Spoon the mixture into the tin and press it down very firmly using the back of a spoon. Cover and leave to cool for at least an hour.
4. Break the chocolate into pieces, put it into a dry bowl and melt it slowly over a saucepan of simmering water. Pour the chocolate over the biscuit base and leave it to set before cutting the tiffin into 16 pieces. Store in an airtight container for up to a week.

## Tea - White, Green and Oolong Tea

*Never heard of it? Well its been around for a very long time and it has been the staple drink of millions of people in China and Japan for thousands of years.*

**Why?**

When it comes to gout, white, green and oolong teas really are the miracle drink. This type of tea is very high in antioxidants as it contains high levels of flavonoids and polyphenols. Five of the flavonoids in green tea are called catechins and these are highly potent antioxidants. One of these, Epigallocatechin Gallette is thought to be twice as powerful as Resveratrol, the polyphenol that is found in grapes. Some research has shown that this type of tea has greater antioxidant capability than Vitamin C and Vitamin E. Green, white and oolong teas also help regulate blood sugar and there is strong evidence that they reduce total cholesterol levels as well as improving the ratio of good HDL to bad LDL cholesterol.

Some of the components in green tea have a similar effect to the NSAID group of drugs, blocking COX-2 enzymes, reducing inflammation and as a consequence limiting the production of free radicals. Some studies have also found that green tea directly inhibits Xanthine Oxidase activity and directly reduces the amount of uric acid that is produced. It is interesting to note that in the United States, the FDA has approved human clinical trials that will study the effects of green tea extract on gout.

All types of tea, irrespective of whether they are green, white, oolong or black, start out as the green leaves of a plant called Camielia Sinensis. The only difference between them is the part of the plant that Is used, where it is grown and how it is processed and fermented.

All green, white and oolong teas are made from loose leaves, leaves that come in a packet not in a paper teabag. They are drunk without milk as the casein in the milk binds to one of the most powerful catechins and this reduces its antioxidant effect. This type of tea is made with water that is below boiling point. The low temperatures that they are made at means that the antioxidant and anti-inflammatory compounds they contain are not damaged during the brewing process. The tea is always made very weak and drunk very fresh, when it has a bright and vibrant colour. As the tea stands its colour changes as it begins to oxidise. Different types of tea contain different amounts of catechins; green and white teas contain between 15% and 30%, oolong between 8% and 20% and black tea between 3% and 10%. You can drink as much of this type of tea as you want and it is an excellent way of keeping yourself well hydrated. Because it is weak it contains very little caffeine.

### How?

You will find green, white and oolong teas in most Chinese supermarkets. You can also buy it on the internet. Its quality varies enormously, as does its price. Just remember that a little goes a long way. Just a few grams are needed to make a large pot and you can obtain two or three 'brews' out of the same leaves.

How you make green, white and oolong tea is critical. Different types of tea need to be made with water at different temperatures. If it is too hot the tea can taste bitter and be unpleasant to drink. Making it with filtered water is a good idea as this brings out the full flavour of the individual tea. How do you make this type of tea? Instructions for making tea is included in the 'More About' section at the end of this book.

### Tip:

Green, White and Oolong teas have beautiful colours so drink them from a glass, not a cup or mug. Try adding some slices of lemon to the tea and then leaving it to cool. Cold tea with lemon makes a very refreshing drink.

## Herbs and Spices

### Why?

As well as adding flavour to your food, herbs and spices also contain large amounts of flavonoids, anthocyanins and phytonutrients. These have powerful antioxidant, anti-inflammatory and medicinal properties. Chilli peppers, rosemary, ginger, bay leaves, cumin, coriander, dill, fennel, garlic, oregano, sage and thyme are all great and their use in cooking as well as medicine goes back a long way. Parsley and chervil have attracted a lot of attention recently as they are both very rich sources of flavonoids, Vitamin C and the beta carotene from which Vitamin A is made. They also contain a very powerful oil called Myristicin which activates an enzyme that works with your body's antioxidant Glutathione in oxidising free radicals. Interestingly, in the middle ages, parsley and chervil were used by the monks as a cure for gout.

### How?

Herbs like basil, parsley, coriander and herb rocket make really good pesto and this is an excellent way of concentrating their health giving properties. The classic Italian paste of gremolatta is basically parsley, lemon zest and garlic and it tastes delicious. When you use pesto you add a completely new dimension to your food. Pesto freezes really well in small pots. Just remember to add any garlic after you have thawed it out, not before, as when it is frozen garlic can develop off flavours that are quite unpleasant.

Herbs and spices have been around for thousands of years and they form a staple part of the diet of many countries. Indian, Asian and North African food all gain their characteristics from herbs and spices. Try chopping them and sprinkling them on your food instead of using sauces and dressing.

### Tip:

Use fresh herbs whenever possible. Dried herbs just don't taste the same. Avoid cooking herbs, especially herbs like basil, dill, coriander, chervil and parsley. It changes their flavour as well as reducing their nutritional benefits. Adding lemon or lime juice preserves their colour even when they are frozen.

What about freezing herbs?

Its fine. In fact its the best way of preserving them as their nutritional value is not damaged and their flavour is only slightly changed.

## Making Pesto

*Pestos are a really good way of using herbs as they enable you to eat the herbs raw and this preserves not only their flavour but also their nutritional value. Adding lemon or lime juice to the pesto preserves its colour by slowing down the rate at which it oxidises.*

*You can use pesto on its own, stirred into yoghurt to make dips and added to vegetables and grains. Mixed with toasted oatmeal or Panko (Japanese) breadcrumbs and optionally with a little grated parmesan or pecorino they make a wonderful crumb topping for fish and vegetables. Just about any herb can be made into pesto. Vegetables like beetroot and semi dried dried tomatoes can also be used. Black and green olives can be processed in exactly the same way to make tapenade.*

*Making pesto is a little time consuming and it is certainly not something you want to do every day. However, the good news is that pesto freezes well and freezing does not destroy any of the pesto's nutritional value. If you are going to make some pesto it is worthwhile making a large batch and freezing it in small portions. Just remember to leave out the garlic as after a few weeks in the freezer it will start to develop a slight musty flavour. You can always add garlic when you thaw the pesto out.*

*How do you freeze pesto? All you need to do is open freeze large spoon fulls on a tray lined with cling film and when the pesto is frozen use some foil to wrap it up into individual parcels. It is also worthwhile investing in some small silicon muffin tins and using these to hold the pesto while it is being frozen.*

## Basil Pesto

*The 'pesto' we all think of as pesto. Like coriander pesto, this is so useful it is worth making it in large quantities. Most recipes for basil pesto use pine nuts but any type of nut will do.*

300g/10½oz basil
100g/3½oz raw cashew nuts
30g/1oz lightly toasted sunflower seeds
10 tbsp olive oil
85g/3oz finely grated parmesan
Crushed garlic to taste

1. Wash and dry the basil and remove any coarse stems.
2. Put the cashew nuts and sunflower seeds into a food processor and grind them.
3. Add the basil to the food processor. You will need to do this in stages as there will be too much basil to go in in one go. When the basil has reduced in volume add the other ingredients and blend well.

## Gremolata

*This is an adaptation of the classical Italian gremolata which is a mixture of very finely chopped parsley and lemon juice. You can use any type of nut but make sure you use flat leaf parsley and not curled parsley as it has a much better flavour.*

| | |
|---|---|
| 250g/9 oz flat leaf parsley | Finely grated zest of a lemon |
| 50g/1¾oz walnuts or pecan nuts | Juice of a lemon |
| 3 tbsp olive oil | Garlic to taste |
| 1 tbsp finely grated parmesan | Salt to taste |

1. Remove any coarse stems from the parsley and then wash and drain it. If necessary dry it in some kitchen paper. Roughly chop it.
2. Grind the walnuts to a fairly fine powder in a food processor. Add all the other ingredients and blend until everything is well mixed into a thick purée.

## Coriander Pesto

*Having coriander pesto in the freezer is really useful, especially when you are making curries.*

| | |
|---|---|
| 175g/6oz coriander leaves and stems | Finely grated zest of a lime |
| 3 tbsp whole almonds with their skins | Juice of a lime |
| 4 tbsp olive oil | 1 tsp finely chopped chilli OR 1 tsp Sambol Oelek |
| Salt to taste | |

1 Wash and dry the coriander. Grind the almonds to a fine powder in a blender or food processor.

2 Roughly chop the coriander and add it with the other ingredients to the almonds in the food processor and blend until fully mixed.

## Carrot, Mango & Coriander Salad

*This is one of the most weird salads ever, but it tastes absolutely delicious and strangely, it goes extremely well with fish, especially salmon, trout and smoked mackerel. You can serve the salad on its own or add chickpeas or beans to make it into a substantial meal.*

*Unfortunately its preparation is somewhat labour intensive as it involves a lot of peeling and slicing. If you can obtain one of the sour green mangos that are grown especially for savoury dishes all the better. Otherwise use the most under ripe mango you can find.*

---

SERVES 4

1 very large green under ripe mango
350g/12oz carrots
1 small red onion peeled and finely chopped
3 - 4 tbsp finely chopped coriander
OR 30g/1oz ready made coriander pesto
Grated zest of 1 lime
Juice of 1 lime
1 tsp Sambol Oelek or chilli paste
1tbsp rice vinegar
1 tbsp Thai fish sauce
1 preserved lemon
3 tbsp lightly toasted pumpkin and sunflower seeds

---

1 First make the salad dressing by mixing together the zest and juice of a lime, the Sambol Oelek ( you can use more than 1 tsp if you like your food spicy), the rice vinegar, the Thai fish sauce and the chopped coriander or pesto.

2 Cut the stone from the mango. Peel the halves of mango and slice the flesh into thin slices. Now cut each of these thin slices into narrow mandolin strips. Put them into a large bowl and pour on the dressing.

3 Peel the carrots and slice them very thinly along their length. Then cut each long slice into narrow very thin mandolin strips.

4 Add the carrots to the mango in the bowl and give everything a good stir.

5 Stir in the finely chopped red onion. You can use spring onions if you prefer but the red onion gives the salad a better colour and more intense flavour.
6 Cut the preserved lemon in half, take out the pips and cut it into very small pieces. Stir it into the salad.
7 Lastly add the toasted seeds. You can use more or less toasted seeds according to taste.
8 Cover and leave the salad for at least half an hour for the flavours to develop.

The salad will keep for up to two days if stored in the fridge but the longer you keep it the more the texture will reduce.

## Thai Carrot Soup

*Yellow Thai curry is made from chillies, turmeric, ginger and garlic. As all of these are strongly anti-inflammatory, a yellow Thai curry or curry soup makes a healthy anti-inflammatory meal. You can buy Thai curry paste on line and in Asian supermarkets. IThis soup freezes well and can be kept in the fridge for up to 2 days.*

---

SERVES 4

1 large white onion finely sliced
1 tbsp olive oil
700g/1 lb 8 oz carrots
1Lt/35 fl oz vegetable stock
100g/3½oz red lentils
1 tbsp yellow Thai curry paste
3 handfuls of coriander finely chopped

---

1 Peel and slice the carrots into 5ml/¼in rounds.

2 Heat the olive oil over a medium heat and add the onion. Sauté for a minute or two. Add the Thai curry paste and the sliced carrots and stir for a minute or two.

3 Add the vegetable stock and the lentils. Turn up the heat and bring the soup to the boil, stirring occasionally to prevent the lentils sticking.

4 Turn the heat to low, cover and simmer for 30 minutes.

5 When you are ready to serve, blitz the soup with a hand blender and stir in half of the chopped coriander. Serve the rest of the coriander in a separate bowl.

## Mussel, Leek & Saffron Soup

*This recipe uses frozen mussels as they take less time to prepare and are widely available in supermarkets. You can also use fresh mussels in their shells if you can get them. If you do use fresh mussels you will need about 1.5Kg/3lb.*

---

SERVES 4

300g/11oz frozen mussel meat, thawed, washed and dried
450g/16oz leeks coarsely chopped
5cm/2in piece white part of a leek cut into match stick size pieces
50ml/2 fl oz white wine OR Noilly Prat (optional)
1 small onion chopped
50g/2oz butter
1tbsp flour
450ml/15 fl oz fish stock OR
450ml/15fl oz vegetable stock and 1Tbsp Thai fish sauce
A large pinch of saffron
50ml/2 fl oz fromage frais or natural unsweetened Greek yoghurt

---

1 Melt the butter in a saucepan and sauté the leeks and onion on a medium heat for 3 - 4 minutes. Be careful not to let them brown.

2 Stir in the flour and cook for 2 minutes. Add the stock and the saffron. If using vegetable stock and Thai fish sauce add the fish sauce just before you serve the soup. Bring everything to the boil, turn down the heat and simmer for 25 - 30 minutes.

3 Use a hand blender to purée the leeks and onion. At this stage you can turn off the heat or leave the soup simmering on a low heat.

4 When you are ready to serve the soup add the mussels, bring the soup to the boil and simmer gently for 5 minutes. Don't overcook the mussels as they will become tough.

5 Just before serving stir in the cream or yoghurt. Ladle the soup into individual bowls and garnish with the slices of leek.

## Chickpea & Cauliflower Curry with Onion Raita

*This is a quick, basic curry sauce that you can use to make any type of curry using vegetables, beans, tofu, fish or seafood. This recipe uses cauliflower and chickpeas. Don't be put off by the long list of ingredients.*

SERVES 4

For the curry sauce
400g/14oz tin chopped tomatoes
1 medium white or red onion finely sliced
2 tbsp olive oil
2 tbsp grated ginger
2 cloves of garlic crushed
1 red chilli finely chopped OR 2 tsp Sambol Oelek
2 tsp ground coriander
1 tsp ground cumin
½ tsp ground fenugreek
½ tsp turmeric
2 tbsp natural unsweetened yoghurt
Juice and finely grated zest of a lemon or lime
2 tbsp coriander very finely chopped
1 medium cauliflower
400g/14oz can chick peas drained and rinsed

Red Onion Raita
1 tsp cumin seeds
1 clove garlic crushed
1 small chilli (optional)
1 large red onion
200ml/7 fl oz natural unsweetened yoghurt
2 tbsp finely chopped coriander
1 tbsp lemon juice

1. First make the Raita. Toast the cumin seeds for 1 – 2 minutes in a dry pan over a moderate heat. Be careful not to let them burn. Lightly crush them using a pestle and mortar.
2. Put the yoghurt into a bowl and add the cumin, garlic and chilli if you are using it.
3. Finely chop the red onion and add it to the yoghurt mixture. Then stir in the chopped coriander and the lemon juice. Cover and put the raita into the fridge.

4 Remove the skins from the tomatoes by covering them with boiling water and leaving them to soak for a minute or two. Drop them into cold water and then peel them. The skins should come off quite easily. Roughly chop the tomatoes. As an alternative you can use a can of chopped tomatoes.

5 Heat the oil in a saucepan and sauté the sliced onion for 2 -3 minutes. Add the tomatoes, cook for a couple of minutes and then stir in the cumin, ground coriander, turmeric, chilli, garlic lime or lemon zest and the ginger. Add 150ml/5fl oz water, bring to the boil, turn down the heat and simmer for 10 minutes while you prepare the cauliflower.

6 Take the outer leaves off of the cauliflower and break the florets into small thumb size pieces. Bring a pan of water to the boil and cook the cauliflower for 3 minutes.

7 Drain the cauliflower and add it with the chickpeas to the curry sauce. Stir in 2 tbsp chopped coriander, the yoghurt and lime or lemon juice. Cook for a 4 -5 minutes until the chickpeas are heated through and the cauliflower is tender.

8 Serve the curry with the Raita in a separate bowl..

## Dairy Products, especially low fat dairy products.

**Why?**

As long ago as the 17th Century the gout patient was told that milk was a good thing to drink. Now science has proved that it really is. Low fat dairy products in the form of both milk and yoghurt are an essential part of a gout diet. But by yoghurt I mean natural unflavoured yoghurt that is not sweetened, not thickened and not pasteurised. It needs to be 'alive and kicking' with acidophilus, bifidus and other probiotics. And you don't need to go out and buy 'probiotic' products as the jury is still out on them. If the yoghurt is alive and not pasteurised and homogenised it will be brimming with healthy bacteria.

All dairy products contain calcium and calcium is one of the few substances known to inhibit the absorption of both HEME and non-HEME iron. When consumed as part of a meal 50mg or less of calcium has little or no effect on the absorption of the iron in the meal but calcium in amounts of 300mg to 600mg does. One cup of skimmed milk contains about 300mg of calcium. One of the objectives of a a gout friendly diet is to reduce the intake of iron, so adding even a modest amount of low fat dairy to a meal will help reduce the amount of iron you absorb from it. Something of a paradox when you consider that breakfast cereals are fortified with iron and most of us have milk or yoghurt with our breakfast cereal!

Low fat dairy products are known to increase the amount of uric acid excreted by the kidneys. This increase in the excretion of uric acid is only slight but every little helps. Around 30% of the uric acid we excrete is eliminated through the digestive tract and this is where live yoghurt has another role. In our digestive tract beneficial bacteria are a naturally occurring phenomenon that is often destroyed by the typical Western diet. Low fat dairy products that are 'alive and kicking' so to speak with bacteria slowly help to repopulate the digestive tract with a healthy spectrum of bacteria and this in turn helps it to eliminate the 30% of uric acid that is excreted there. Probiotic bacteria also help reduce inflammation. We have hundreds of different types of bacteria in our digestive tract and there is strong evidence to suggest that some of the 'good' bacteria have a positive impact on our immune system, particularly in correcting deficiencies.

But take care. A surprisingly large number of people are allergic or have a level of intolerance to dairy products. If you are one of these, low fat diary will simply fuel the inflammation that already exists so avoid them like the plague and use a probiotic supplement instead. You could also try sheep or goat milk products which are often more easily tolerated.

### How?

You can drink milk and eat yoghurt at any time. Yoghurt makes a really good start to the day. Add your own fruit, without sugar, and if needs be the fruit can be frozen. Use yoghurt to make smoothies, again these can be frozen. You can use yoghurt for dressings instead of mayonnaise and flavoured with lime zest and herbs it makes a wonderful addition stirred into soup. Try mixing it with grated cucumber, carrot or mint and using it as a dip for vegetables.

Cottage cheese, curd cheese, 'hard' cheese and cream are all good, provided you remember that cream and hard cheese contains a lot of fat and are therefore high in calories. By cheese I mean real cheese that has a rind and tastes of something, not the processed dyed stuff that comes in orange or yellow slabs. Camembert and blue cheeses like Roquefort and Stilton are all good. If you can obtain it try goats or sheep's cheese. They both have a very pronounced flavour so you eat much less of it. Hard cheeses like parmesan and pecorino have intensely strong flavours and a little grated over your food goes a long way. Eat cheese with celery and apple as this means you are consuming saturated fats with antioxidants. Have a go at making your own ice cream but use stevia instead of sugar. Better still make frozen yoghurt. Its just as good as ice cream and much better for you.

## Cranachan

*A traditional Scottish dessert made from toasted oatmeal. The oatmeal is soaked overnight in whisky and honey and then mixed with soft cheese and raspberries. Most recipes you see today do not soak the oatmeal and they use whipped cream instead of the cheese. This recipe uses half fromage frais and half thick Greek yoghurt instead of the cream but you could also use a soft low fat soft cheese like Ricotta or Quark. The whisky gives the dessert it's characteristic flavour. Whether you use Whiskey and how much you use is a matter of personal taste.*

SERVES 4

300ml/10 fl oz (½pt) fromage frais
300ml/10 fl oz (½pt) thick unsweetened Greek yoghurt
85g/3 oz flaked oats that have been toasted golden brown
3 tbsp Whisky
3 tbsp runny honey
450g/1lb raspberries
Toasted flaked almonds to garnish

1 Mix 2 tbsp of the honey and 2 tbsp of the whiskey with the toasted oatmeal and leave it to soak.. How long you soak it for is a matter of taste. The longer it soaks the softer it becomes.
2 Beat the fromage frais and yoghurt together until they are thoroughly blended and then stir in the remaining honey and whisky.
3 Crush half of the raspberries lightly with a fork and stir them into the yoghurt mixture.
4 Put a layer of whole raspberries into the bottom of 4 desert glasses. Put in a layer of the yoghurt mixture and then a layer of the oatmeal. Continue until you have used all the raspberries. Finish with a layer of yoghurt. Garnish with the toasted flaked almonds before serving.

## Russian Raspberry Pudding

*A simple very easy recipe that can be eaten hot or cold. Fresh raspberries are best but you can also use frozen raspberries. The recipe uses a small amount of sugar. You can substitute Stevia or another artificial sweetener if you wish. When it is hot, straight from the oven, this recipe smells delicious and I think it is the best way to eat raspberries.*

SERVES 4

450g/1lb raspberries
2 tbsp caster sugar.
150ml/5 fl oz (¼ pt) fromage frais
150ml/5 fl oz (¼ pt) thick unsweetened Greek yoghurt
2 large free range eggs
1 tbsp flour
1 tbsp Demerera sugar

Pre heat the oven to 150°C/ 300°F/Gas 2

1 Put the raspberries into a greased gratin dish and sprinkle then with 1 tbsp of caster sugar. Put the dish into the middle of the oven and leave them to heat through for 10 minutes.

2 Beat the fromage frais, yoghurt, eggs, flour and remaining tbsp caster sugar together. Pour this over the raspberries and sprinkle on the demerera sugar. Put the raspberries back into the oven on the top shelf. Leave the oven on the same temperature.

3 Cook for about 45 minutes until the top is light golden brown and firm to touch

## Eggs

### Why?

Eggs are an excellent source of protein and essential fatty acids. In fact when it comes to nutrients there is very little that eggs do not have. However, in order to ensure that you have a healthy ratio of Omega-3 to Omega-6 make sure you buy free range eggs from hens that spend their life running around in a field. The nutritional content of a free range egg, especially its Omega-3 content, is totally different to an egg from a hen that is kept in a battery farm. You do not need to buy Omega-3 enriched eggs either. All this means is that the poor battery hen has been fed on fish meal, the eggs from the happy hens will have just as much Omega-3.

*Eggs contain iron and a gout friendly diet avoids iron rich foods?*

Yes eggs do contain iron. A large egg contains about 1mg of iron which is quite a lot when you consider how small an egg is. But eggs also contain a phosphoprotein called phosvita and this binds to iron and reduces its bioavailability. One boiled egg can reduce the absorption of not only the iron in the egg but also the other iron in a meal by as much as 25%.

*Eggs are bad for me, they contain a large amount of cholesterol?*

Yes its true, they do contain a large amount of cholesterol. A large boiled eggs weighs around 50 grams and it contains around 200mg of cholesterol. The same 50 gram portion of lean beef contains around 40mg. It's the same old myth about saturated fats. Eggs contain a lot of healthy things as well as cholesterol. If they form part of a diet that is rich in antioxidants, vitamins, minerals and fibre they are fine.

### How?

Boil or poach them, scramble them lightly in butter or use them in an omelette. Just avoid frying them. Mixed with vegetables like spinach, courgettes, peppers and butter nut squash they make great Spanish tortillas.

## Egg Soubise

*Soubise is a thick creamy sauce that is traditionally made with onions and cream. This recipe is quick and easy to prepare. It can be served with any type of vegetable or a simple salad. Without the boiled eggs the soubise will keep in the fridge for a couple of days. It can also be frozen. You can if you wish add some cooked mussels to the soubise just before you put it into the oven. This works particularly well if the soubise is made from leeks instead of onions. The large amount of onions used in this recipe makes this a good anti-inflammatory dish.*

SERVES 4

750g/1lb 10oz white onions sliced
1 tbsp butter
3 tbsp milk
Finely grated zest and juice of ½ lemon
2 bay leaves
2 tbsp Japanese panko breadcrumbs
300ml/10 fl oz (½pt) fromage frais or Greek style natural unsweetened yoghurt
6 large free range eggs that have been hard boiled.
Crushed black pepper to taste

1 Heat the butter in a saucepan and gently sauté the onions over a medium heat for 5 minutes. Stir in the milk, the bay leaves and lemon zest, cover the saucepan, reduce the heat to low and simmer the onions for 30 minutes until they are soft. Leave them to cool slightly.
2 Pre heat the oven to 180°C/ 350°F/Gas 4
3 Peel the eggs and cut them in half. Put them cut side down either in individual dishes or in a single layer in a baking dish.
4 Remove the bay leaves and add the yoghurt, crushed black pepper and lemon juice to the onions. Purée them using a hand blender. Stir in the breadcrumbs and pour the purée over the eggs. Bake for 20 minutes.

## Eggs in a Coconut Curry Sauce

*A quick and easy way to serve eggs. For a healthy low carbohydrate option serve the curry with cauliflower 'rice'.*

SERVES 4

8 large free range eggs
1 large white onion finely sliced
1 tbsp olive oil
1 small chilli finely chopped OR 2 tsp Sambol Oelek or chilli paste
2 cloves of garlic crushed
400ml/14fl oz can coconut milk
3 large tomatoes cut into quarters
2 tbsp finely grated ginger
1 tsp turmeric
2 tsp ground coriander
½ tsp ground green cardamom
3 tbsp fresh coriander chopped
1 large cauliflower, white only

1. Sauté the sliced onion in the olive oil for 5 minutes. Add the garlic, chilli, turmeric, cardamom and ground coriander. Cook for a minute or two and then add the coconut milk, grated ginger and tomatoes. Bring to the boil, reduce the heat and leave the sauce to simmer while you cook the eggs and cauliflower.
2. Boil the eggs for 12 minutes. Peel them, cut them in half and add them to the curry sauce.
3. Break the cauliflower into florets and cook it in boiling water for 3 to 4 minutes until it is just tender. Drain it and use a potato ricer or hand blender to mash it into a rough grainy texture.
4. Sprinkle the chopped coriander onto the egg curry just before serving with the cauliflower 'rice'.

## Omelettes

*A classic omelette is quick and easy to make. You can fill it with a variety of different ingredients; sliced mushrooms that have been lightly sautéed, baby spinach leaves wilted with some chopped tomato and chilli, a handful of chives and mixed herbs and, strange as it may sound, a few spoonfuls of petite pois mixed with some wilted lettuce and lemon juice. The combinations are endless.*

*The technique is simple and success depends mainly on having a frying pan that is the right size for the number of eggs; if the pan is too big the omelette will be thin and tough, if it is too small it will be spongy and thick.*

*Eggs are inflammatory? Yes they are but only mildly and by adding just a tiny amount of chilli, cayenne pepper, garlic or turmeric you can balance out their inflammatory effect. Serve them with broccoli or a salad of baby spinach leaves and they provide a healthy nutritious anti-inflammatory meal.*

## Sardine Omelette

*A strange combination but one that tastes really good and it is quick and easy to prepare. You can use any type of tinned oily fish to make this. Sardines work particularly well but make sure you use sardine fillets that have been canned in olive oil not sunflower oil.*

SERVES 2

120g/4¼ oz sardine fillets in olive oil
5 large free range eggs
4 spring onions sliced OR half red onion finely chopped
Half finely chopped red chilli or ½ tsp chilli paste
1 large or 2 small tomatoes finely sliced.

1. Pour 1 tablespoon of the olive oil from the sardines into an omelette pan and drain the rest away. Break up the sardine fillets into large flakes.
2. Whisk the eggs until the whites and yolks are combined. Stir in the onions, the chopped chilli or chilli paste and the sardines.
3. Heat the grill on high.
4. Heat the oil in the omelette pan over a medium heat and pour in the eggs, tipping the eggs from side to side so that they are evenly spread.
5. Using a fork gently draw the edges of the egg towards the centre of the pan and let the liquid egg run to the edges. Keep doing this until the omelette is almost set but still moist on top.
6. Turn off the heat and put a layer of sliced tomatoes over the top of the omelette. Put it under the grill for 2 – 3 minutes until the tomatoes are heated through. Serve immediately with some green vegetables or a green salad

## Tortilla, Frittata & Kuku

*A Kuku is a sort of solid unfolded omelette that contains vegetables and herbs. It is more like a Spanish tortilla or an Italian Frittata than a traditional omelette which should be lightly cooked and only just set in the centre. Kukus' originated in ancient Persia. It is hardly surprising that there is a similarity between the tortilla and the frittata as the kuku was brought to Spain by the Arabs and the spice traders brought it to Italy.*

*You can basically use more or less any vegetable to make kukus, tortillas and frittatas. Just make sure the ingredients are freshly cooked otherwise the finished dish will have a stale leftover taste. You can serve tortillas, frittatas and kukus hot or cold, as a main course, cut in slices for a picnic or cut into small squares as canapés. They make an excellent breakfast dish and they will keep for up to 2 days in a fridge.*

*Recipes for these types of egg dishes vary. Some add baking powder and some add flour, most are cooked slowly in a covered non stick frying pan. Whichever recipe you use and whichever way you choose to cook it, this type of egg dish provides a nutritious meal that is quick and easy to prepare.*

*Egg dishes of this type have a reputation of being a bit 'dried up'. Adding a small amount of cream, yoghurt or fromage frais helps prevent this. One thing you do need when making a tortilla, frittata or kuku is a high quality non stick frying pan, preferably one with a lid. If you can find one with a metal handle that you can put into the oven all the better as the easiest and fail safe way of cooking a tortilla or frittata is to start the process on the hob and then finish it in the oven.*

## Broccoli & Brie Frittata

*You can make this with any type of broccoli and use either brie, Camembert or a soft goats log. You will need a 24cm/10 inch non stick frying pan that can go into the oven. Adding a small amount of yoghurt is optional but it does help to soften the tortilla and prevent it from becoming too hard.*

---

SERVES 4

6 large free range eggs
3 tbsp natural unsweetened yoghurt (optional)
1 tbsp olive oil
400g/14oz tender stem or purple sprouting broccoli
175g/6oz brie or goats log
½ tsp garlic powder
¼ tsp ground turmeric
2 tbsp toasted pine nuts

---

Pre heat the oven to 180°C/ 350°F/Gas 4

1 Cook the broccoli for 3 minutes. Drain and put to one side to cool a little.
2 Cut the cheese into 1cm/½ in pieces.
3 Whisk the eggs and yoghurt in a large bowl with the turmeric and garlic powder. Season to taste with salt and pepper. Mix the broccoli, cheese and pine nuts into the eggs.
4 Heat the frying pan with 1 tsp olive oil over a medium heat and add the eggs, broccoli and cheese. Cook for 5 minutes then cover it and put the pan into the oven. Cook for 20 minutes.
5 Pre heat the grill to high. Take the frying pan out of the oven, remove the lid and pop it under the grill until the top of the tortilla is set. Serve at once.

## Vegetable Torte

*This is somewhere between a pastry-less quiche and a terrine. You can make it with more or less any vegetables that you have available. The torte will keep for up to 2 days in the fridge but it will not freeze.*

SERVES 6 - 8

250g/9oz courgette
250g/9oz cauliflower broken into small florets
70g/2½oz fine French beans
1 medium white onion finely chopped
1 tbsp olive oil
2 cloves of garlic crushed
2 finely chopped preserved lemons
2 tbsp chopped basil
5 tbsp finely grated parmesan
200g/7oz feta
350g/12oz silken tofu
4 large free range eggs

Pre heat the oven to 160°C/325°F/Gas 3

1. Grease a 20cm/8 in cake tin and dust the inside with finely grated parmesan.
2. Sauté the onion and garlic in the olive oil over a medium heat for 5 minutes. Stir it occasionally, do not let it brown. Put to one side.
3. Top and tail the French beans and boil them for 3 – 4 minutes. Drain and refresh in cold water.
4. Put the cauliflower into a large microwave bowl, add 3 tablespoons of water, cover and cook on full power for 3 minutes. Take the cauliflower out and put it to one side.
5. If the courgettes are large cut them in half lengthways and cut each half into 5mm/¼ in slices. Put the sliced courgette and the mange tout into the microwave bowl, cover and cook for 3 minutes. Leave to cool.
6. Cut half of the feta into small 5mm/¼ in dice. Put the rest into a bowl with the tofu, eggs, chopped basil and the parmesan and blend everything together using a hand blender.

7 Stir in the onions, the vegetables, the chopped preserved lemons and diced feta.

8 Pour the mixture into the prepared cake tin, cover loosely with foil and bake in the centre of the oven for 45 minutes. Take the foil off and cook for another 15 minutes. Turn off the oven and leave the torte to cool before taking it out.

## Not Quite An Arnold Bennett Omelette

*Traditionally an Arnold Bennett omelette is an omelette for 2 people that is topped with smoked haddock and a creamy béchamel sauce. This is a more substantial version that uses salmon or trout and courgette to turn the omelette into a meal for 4 people. You can use any cut of salmon or trout to make this.*

---

SERVES 4

2 courgettes weighing about 400g/14oz
1 tsp dried dill
6 large free range eggs
1 tsp olive oil
350g/12oz skinned and boned salmon
300ml/10 fl oz (½pt) natural Greek style unsweetened yoghurt
1 tsp cornflour
50g/1¾oz finely grated parmesan or other hard cheese
Salt and pepper to taste

---

You will need a 26cm/10 in non stick frying pan or chefs pan with a lid to make this.

Pre heat the oven to 200°C/ 400°F/Gas 5

1 Wash and dry the salmon and cut it into 1cm/½ in pieces.
2 Whisk one of the eggs, 1 tsp dried dill and 1 tsp cornflour into the yoghurt and put to one side.
3 Whisk the other 5 eggs in a large bowl and season to taste with salt and pepper.
4 Coarsely grate the courgette and mix it into the eggs.
5 Heat the frying pan with 1 tsp olive oil over a medium heat and add the pieces of salmon. Cover and cook them for 5 minutes. By this time the fish should be just set and translucent. Use a slotted spoon to remove it from the pan and put it to one side.
6 Add the egg and courgette mixture to the pan and cook for 5 minutes over a moderate heat. Put on the lid and transfer the pan to the oven. Cook for 10 minutes.

7 Reduce the oven to 180°C/ 350°F/Gas 4

8 Take the frying pan out of the oven, remove the lid and put the salmon on top of the 'omelette' in a single layer. Pour the yoghurt and egg mixture on top. Put the pan back in the oven without the lid and bake for 10 minutes.

9 Pre heat the grill to high. Take the frying pan out of the oven, sprinkle on the grated cheese and pop it under the grill until the cheese has melted.

Serve with green vegetables or a green salad.

## Tofu and Soya Bean Products

*.... but only in the form of bean curd, Tempeh and miso. Not in the form of 'mock' or 'imitation' meat or when it is added as 'textured vegetable protein' to make vegie burgers, pad out processed meat products and make junk food like soya cheese and ice cream.*

*Why? The soya used is almost always a bye-product of the manufacture of soya bean oil and it is very heavily processed. It is often made from soya beans that have been grown using questionable farming methods and it also contains residual products left over from the oil manufacturing process and these are far from being healthy.*

**Why?**

Tofu, bean curd and Tempeh are amazing products that are high in protein, low in fat, low in calories, easy to digest and cheap. They also contain all of the eight essential amino acids as well as Vitamin A and Vitamin B. Tempeh is a particularly valuable source of Vitamin B12.

Tofu in the form of bean curd originated in China over one thousand years ago. Originally it was the poor man's protein but when one of the Emperors started eating it it became fashionable and soon it was more or less a staple food. It has remained so ever since.

Tofu and bean curd is made from dried soya beans in a 'process' that is fairly similar to cheese making. The soya beans used can be black, green or white. The whole beans are soaked and then ground into a paste. A coagulant is added and the solid 'curds' then separated out. Tempeh is made from whole beans that are soaked, fermented and then inoculated with a culture that binds them together into a solid cake. Even though both tofu and tempeh are processed foods they are very close to the dried soya beans they are made from. If you look at the label you will see soya beans, water and in the case of bean curd, coagulants such as calcium sulphite (gypsum), nigari (magnesium chlorate) or GDL (delta glucano lactose). They may sound horrendous but these coagulants have been used to make the product for hundreds of years.

There has been and still is a lot of controversy about tofu and soya bean products generally. To a large extent this is because they contain plant oestrogens and phytic acid. However, it is easy to lose sight of the fact that they are a food that has been consumed by people in the Far East for thousands of years and most of the people who eat them today are far healthier than their Western counterparts. The Okinawans in Japan are some of the world's healthiest and long lived people and, together with fish, tofu is one of their staple foods.

**How**

Tofu comes in different textures and colours in the form of bean curd. Together with tempeh it is the meat, eggs and cheese to committed vegetarians. To others it is 'Terrible Tofu', 'Tasteless Tofu' or 'Rubbery squares that look awful'. You rarely hear a good word said about it. However, what it looks like and what it tastes like depend on how it is cooked. One of the great things about soya bean products are they they absorb the flavours of the things they are cooked with.

Tofu, bean curd and tempeh can be steamed, poached in a sauce, lightly sautéed, crumbled into vegetables and even puréed to make dips and salad dressings. Dare I say it, but they can also be marinated and then roasted, baked or fried. Silken tofu makes really good 'cheesecakes' and it provides a highly nutritious base for terrines. It is particularly valuable for people who are lactose intolerant.

Tofu is a controversial food. If you google it you will get a raft of conflicting information and much of this is mis-information. However, it is not a 'miracle' health food, neither is it something dangerous that should be avoided. Whatever the truth, tofu and bean curd products are made from beans and, unlike meat, these have not been subjected to intensive farming methods and injected with hormones and antibiotics. As such they provide a valuable alternative source of protein.

## Carrot, Lentil & Pistachio Loaf

*This recipe uses silken tofu to add additional protein to the lentils. The loaf makes a substantial family meal. It can be made in advance, cooked and then warmed up when needed. It does not freeze well once it is cooked but it can be frozen uncooked.*

SERVES 4 - 6

1 large free range egg
50g/1½oz finely chopped coriander
OR 30g/1oz coriander pesto
2 tbsp grated ginger
200g/6½oz red lentils
400g/13oz carrots, peeled and finely grated
50g/1½oz shelled pistachio nuts
350g/12oz silken tofu
1 clove garlic crushed (optional)

Grease and line a 1.4Lt/2 ½ pt loaf tin and heat the oven to 180°C/ 350°F/Gas 4

1 Wash the lentils and pick them over carefully to make sure there is no grit in them. Drain them in a sieve, put them into a saucepan and add 350ml/12 fl oz of cold water. Bring them to the boil, cover, turn down the heat to low and cook very slowly for 20 minutes. The lentils should be just cooked and the water absorbed. Leave them to cool a little.

2 Put the grated carrot and the grated ginger into a microwave bowl. Cover and cook on full power for 5 minutes. Take off the cover and leave to cool a little.

3 Drain the tofu and put it into a large bowl with the egg, Use a hand blender to blend it thoroughly into a thick paste.

4 Add the grated carrot, the cooked lentils, the garlic, pistachio nuts and the chopped coriander to the tofu and egg mixture. Give it a good stir and put it into the loaf tin and bake for half an hour. Turn the oven down to 160°C/ 325°F/Gas 3 and bake for another 30 minutes. Leave for 5 to 10 minutes before serving.

## Miso, Tofu & Tahini Dip

*Silken tofu can be made into dips and it is a very useful ingredient for people who are unable to eat dairy products. This is an interesting dip that can be served on its own, with crudités or used as a dressing for vegetables and noodles. It freezes well but leave out the garlic if you are going to freeze it and add it later.*

---

350g/12oz silken tofu
2 cloves garlic crushed
2 tbsp white miso
8 tbsp Tahini
Juice of 1 lemon OR 2 limes
3 tbsp light soy sauce
Crushed black pepper to taste
4 tbsp finely sliced chives

---

Put everything together in a bowl and blend with a hand blender until you have a smooth paste. Stir in half of the chives, put the dip into a serving bowl and sprinkle the remaining chives on top.

## Butter and Other Saturated Fats

*- but only in moderation. They are high energy foods.*

### Why?

It is a fact that any fat or oil can become harmful when it is oxidised. The more saturated the fat is the less likely it is to oxidise. You can avoid the potential disease causing effects of fats either by not eating them or protecting them from oxidation by also eating plenty of antioxidants. Not consuming them is the conventional approach. Hence why we have been told for years that saturated fats are bad for us. However, this approach has the potential of depriving our body of essential fatty acids that are needed to help us build our body's antioxidant defences as well as a large number of hormones and Vitamin D. It also takes a lot of the enjoyment out of eating.

With the exception of people who are genetically predisposed to developing high levels of cholesterol, it is perfectly safe for us to consume moderate amounts of saturated fats, provided they form part of a healthy diet and are consumed with plenty of vegetables and fruit. In other words large amounts of antioxidants. A fact most people are unaware of is that the group of cholesterol lowering drugs called Statins have an antioxidant activity as well as an anti-platelet activity that is similar to that of antioxidant vitamins. The beneficial effects of this group of drugs stems as much from these properties as it does to their ability to directly reduce cholesterol. Saturated fats and cholesterol are not in themselves bad. It is the lack of antioxidants and high levels of free radicals that make good cholesterol bad.

### How?

Eat and enjoy but only in moderation. Eat only pure butter, not spreadable homogenised butter or butter that is mixed with vegetable oils and trans fats. Remember, fat is a high energy food. One gram of fat contains about 9kcals of energy. One gram of carbohydrate contains about 4kcal. Use a teaspoon as a means of portion control. You will be surprised to learn that one teaspoon contains about 8 grams of butter and as butter is 80% fat this amounts to 50 calories. Where ever you use margarine replace it with butter. Butter oxidises much less than polyunsaturated oils when it is heated but be mindful of your cooking methods. Irrespective of what type of fat you use fried foods are not a particularly healthy option.

*Are there other saturated fats?*

A clarified form of butter called ghee has been used for cooking in India for centuries. Interestingly as it contains virtually no lactose it is fine for people who are otherwise lactose intolerant. It has a slightly nutty flavour and you can usually find it in Asian food stores. Also goose fat and dare I say it good old fashioned beef fat or tallow, coconut oil and things like lard are making a comeback.

What about the Omega 6 PUFA's in lard and goose fat? Well some people think that it is bad but in reality it needs to be put into perspective as the amount of Omega 6 PUFA's is not very different to the amount found in olive oil. Irrespective of whether it comes from grass fed or grain fed animals the amount of Omega 6 PUFA's is still far lower than the Omega 6 found in polyunsaturated vegetable oils and trans fats.

For sixty years conventional medical advice has been that saturated fats cause heart disease. Even now we are told over and over again that this is the case. An editorial in the BMJ "*From the heart. Saturated fat is not the major issue*", attracted a lot of media attention. It stated that it was time to bust the myth that saturated fat causes heart disease.

Reducing saturated fat intake reduces the number of large buoyant (Type A) LDL particles. However, it is the small, dense (Type B) LDL particles that are implicated in heart disease and these only respond to reduction in carbohydrate consumption, not the reduction of saturated fat. A high carbohydrate and high sugar diet raises your risk of heart disease by increasing the number of dense Type B LDL particles and it is also a major factor in the development of metabolic syndrome, a medical condition that goes hand in hand with gout.

Our bodies need saturated fats. We just need to remember that like all fats and oils they are high in calories and should only be eaten in moderate amounts as part of a balanced diet.

## Olive Oil

### Why?

Olive oil is a mono unsaturated oil that has been around for a long time. It contains large amounts of oleic acid and this is the most commonly found monounsaturated fatty acid in our bodies. Oleic acid is also found in oils from almonds, pecans, cashews, peanuts and avocados.

Olive oil contains 75% oleic acid, 13% saturated fat in the form of palmitic acid, 10% Omega-6 and 2% Omega-3 and this makes it a very healthy oil. It is also rich in polyphenols which have antioxidant, anti-inflammatory, anti-clotting and anti-bacterial properties. Olive oil is an oil that has been widely used in Mediterranean, North African and Middle Eastern cooking for hundreds if not thousands of years so it has withstood the test of time. There is no doubt that it is the safest vegetable oil you can use, provided of course that it is consumed in sensible amounts. At the end of the day olive oil is a fat, and very pure fat at that. One gram weighs in so to speak at just under 9kcal, so for a teaspoon think 40kcal and for a tablespoon think 120kcal.

### How?

Always use 'cold pressed' olive oil and keep it in a dark bottle or in the fridge. Simply use it everywhere you would otherwise have used polyunsaturated oils but don't fry with it. Instead lightly sauté your food or bake it a moderate temperature. As with all oils, applying a high heat will oxidise it and create damaging free radicals. Olive oil also makes great salad dressings mixed with lemon juice and herbs.

## Chocolate and Cocoa

*Or rather the dark, bitter 90% plus cocoa solid chocolate with no sugar. Most definitely not the 50% or less cocoa solid chocolate 'candy' bar that is packed full of high fructose corn syrup, vegetable oils and loads of other things that are most definitely not good for you. This type of confectionery does not cure gout it causes it.*

### Why?

High quality, high cocoa mass chocolate and cocoa powder without sugar are possibly the only real 'miracle food' when it comes to gout. But, and its a very big but, not all chocolate and cocoa powder are created equal. The word chocolate really does mean the 90% plus stuff with little or no sugar and as a consequence it tastes very bitter. This type of chocolate is a potent source of antioxidants and it is rich in the polyphenols and flavonoids that help reduce inflammation. Depending on the way it is processed cocoa can contain up to 10% of its weight in flavonoids. The flavonoid group contains the same catechins, epicatechins and proanthocyanidins that are found in green and white tea. These work with the polyphenols to help suppress the inflammatory response because they act as COX-2 inhibitors, working in much the same way as non steroidal anti-inflammatory drugs, NSAID's.

Chocolate is made from seeds or beans that are formed inside pods of fruit on a plant called Theobroma Cacao, or "Food of the Gods", that is native to Central and South America. It has been used as a drink by the indigenous population of South America for hundreds of years, and this drink was known for its health giving properties. However, it is very different to the cocoa drink we know today.

The beans of the cacao tree are extremely bitter, in fact they are so bitter they are inedible. They go through a process of fermentation, sprouting, drying, cleaning and roasting that brings out their flavour. At the end of this process they are ground and the cocoa butter they contain extracted and sold as a separate product. Around 55% of the cocoa bean is cocoa butter. This contains oleic acid and a high proportion of saturated fats that are derived from stearic and palmitic acids. Unlike the cocoa mass it contains very few flavonoids. The cocoa mass or cocoa powder that is left is what we know as cocoa. With most chocolate, fats and oils that are not particularly healthy are put back into the cocoa mass together with sugar, High Fructose Corn Syrup, milk, bulking agents and flavouring to make what we know as chocolate. In 'healthy' chocolate the cocoa butter is put back in with just enough sugar to make the chocolate edible.

As with all things that are heated the flavonoids and antioxidants in the beans are damaged during the roasting process. Most chocolate is heated to very high temperatures, so not only are the flavonoids and antioxidants significantly reduced in numbers, other damage causing substances like AGE's are also produced. Only a few companies process cocoa slowly at low temperatures so retaining many of the health giving benefits of the chocolate.

### How?

The first thing is to find a good source of healthy chocolate or sugar free cocoa powder and this is easier said than done. Medicinal grade chocolate or high quality baking chocolate or cocoa is an option but as this is very difficult to come by most of us have to be pragmatic and make compromises. Go for 90% plus cocoa solids with little or no added sugar. If you have access to the internet go online and see what you can find. Experiment with using cocoa as a drink using stevia as a sweetener. But remember, chocolate contains quite a lot of fat and this means calories, so eat or drink it only in small quantities.

## Chocolate Crunch Biscuits

*This recipe is a war time recipe that uses no eggs and very little sugar and fat. The biscuits are very easy to make and taste surprisingly good.*

Make about 16

2 heaped tbsp unrefined dark Muscavado sugar

2 tbsp cocoa powder

50g/1¾oz butter

3 tbsp water

½ tsp vanilla extract (optional)

150g/5½oz flaked oatmeal

You will need a 20cm/8 in square tin, preferably silicon bakeware, .

Pre heat the oven to 160°C/ 325°F/Gas 3. If the baking tin you are using is metal grease the bottom of the tin really well or line it with baking parchment.

1 Put the butter, sugar, water and cocoa powder into a medium size saucepan and melt the butter over a gentle heat. Stir it well to remove any lumps of sugar and cook, stirring once or twice over a very low heat to 'cook' the cocoa powder and remove the raw cocoa taste.

2 Turn off the heat and add the flaked oatmeal to the butter and cocoa. Mix thoroughly. The mix will be quite dry and become harder to work as it cools. Put it into the prepared tin and using the back of a spoon press it down firmly.

3 Cook for 20 minutes until it is firm to touch. Take it out of the oven and put to one side to cool a little.

4 When it is cool enough to handle put the biscuit onto a chopping board and use a sharp knife to cut it into 16 pieces.

## Chocolate Brownies

*Use any type of nut to make these, almonds, pecan nuts, hazelnuts and walnuts all work. You can serve the brownies on their own or with fromage frais. You will need a 20cm/8 in square cake tin.*

Makes 12 – 16

100g/3½oz nuts
100g/3½oz butter
100g/3½oz 70% or 85% chocolate
2 large free range eggs beaten
40g/1½ oz wholegrain spelt
40g/1½ oz polenta
3 tbsp dark unrefined Muscavado sugar
2 tsp baking powder

Pre heat the oven to 180°C/ 350°F/Gas 4 and grease and line the cake tin.

1. Roughly chop the nuts and toast them for 4 minutes. Take them out and give them a stir, put them back in and toast them for another 4 minutes. Take them out of the oven and put them to one side while you prepare other ingredients.
2. Turn the oven down to 160°C/ 325°F/Gas 3.
3. Break the chocolate into a dry bowl, add the butter and sugar and put the bowl over a saucepan of gently simmering water until the chocolate and butter have melted. Stir until the mixture is smooth. Turn off the heat.
4. Put the spelt, polenta, baking powder and nuts into a bowl. Add the melted chocolate and the beaten eggs and mix well. Spoon into the prepared tin, smooth over the surface and bake for 25 - 30 minutes. The brownies will feel slightly springy in the middle when they are cooked. Leave to cool before cutting into 12 or 16 pieces.

## Water; good old fashioned 'Adams Ale'

**Why?**

If you have gout you are 'crispy'. You are not drinking enough water, or to be more precise, you are not drinking enough water for 'you' and that could well be entirely different to the amount somebody else needs to drink. Your urine needs to be light in colour and clear.

When you read about gout and drinking water, eight glasses a day keeps cropping up. Where this figure comes from is anyone's guess, but you do need to keep yourself well hydrated. You will learn by trial and error how much this needs to be. Contrary to much of what you read you do not need to add bicarbonate of soda to the water. Just plain water will do. Yes there are questions about the quality of tap water. It is up to you whether you buy bottled water or invest in a water filter or water purifier.

**Tip:**

Remember coffee and alcohol dehydrate you so take a glass of water with your coffee or glass of wine. Put soup onto the menu. In fact put it at the top of the menu. Soup as part of your meal will help hydrate you and because it helps to fill you up you will probably eat less.

Celery and fruit contain quite a lot of water so make sure you include them in your diet.

If you are bored with water make your own lemonade from lemons or limes. You can use stevia if you find it too sharp without sugar. It freezes well and you can add dried elder flowers and black currents for variety.

# The 'Not Quite So Good'

## Whole grains

*In the form of Oatmeal, Quinoa, Millet, Buckwheat, Bulgar wheat, Spelt and Barley*

**Why?**

While these are still carbohydrate foods, they are complex carbohydrates with a lower glycemic index than refined carbohydrates like rice and potatoes. This means that they stay in your stomach for longer and take longer to metabolise. As a consequence they release their glucose much more slowly. This results in insulin being better regulated as it is released slowly in line with the release of the glucose. When you eat complex carbohydrates you also feel 'fed' for much longer. Because these types of complex carbohydrates are essentially the complete seed of a plant they contain a surprising amount of vitamins and minerals and they also contain a lot of fibre. While the overall calorie content of these whole grains is relatively high their calorie to fat ratios are different and overall they contain less carbohydrate than the refined carbohydrates most of us consume.

As with so many other things not all wholegrains are created equal. Some are much better than others. Oatmeal, quinoa, millet and buckwheat, (a seed that has nothing to do with wheat) are in reality much better than bulgar wheat, spelt and barley as all wheat products, irrespective of whether they are wholegrain or complex, are mildly to moderately inflammatory, especially when consumed in large amounts. One of the objectives of the gout diet is to reduce inflammation and inflammatory markers.

### Oats in the form of oatmeal

Some people regard oatmeal as a sort of 'superfood'. Notwithstanding this it provides high levels of fibre, low levels of fat and high levels of protein. One cup, or 125 grams, contains only 130 kcals and it contains much less gluten than wheat.

Why do some people regard it as a superfood? There are quite a few reasons.

- Oatmeal contains high levels of magnesium and as magnesium is needed for the production of insulin, it is claimed that it helps stabilise blood sugar and as a consequence reduce the risk of type 2 diabetes developing.
- It removes bad cholesterol and protects good cholesterol from being converted into bad cholesterol. Many studies have shown that a fibre called beta-glucan that is unique to oatmeal has a beneficial effect on cholesterol levels. It also contains an antioxidant called avenanthranmide that again is unique to oatmeal and this prevents free radicals from damaging LDL cholesterol and converting it into bad cholesterol.
- It contains plant lignans which are converted in the digestive tract into mammalian lignans. One of these is called enterolactone and it is thought to protect against heart disease and some cancers.

The larger the 'flake' the less processed the oatmeal is, the more nutrients it retains and the slower it is to digest. You can make your own Muesli with oatmeal by adding nuts and dried fruit, and good old fashioned porridge has stood the test of time. You can also make muesli bars and flapjacks and 'pin head' oatmeal makes wonderful oatcakes.

## Quinoa

Quinoa, pronounced "keen-wah" has been eaten for 5,000 years by the people of South America. It is not a grain but a seed from a vegetable that is closely related to Swiss Chard. It is a complex carbohydrate with a low glycemic index.

Quinoa contains twice as much protein as other cereal grains. At 18% its protein content is about the same as milk. The protein it contains is also a 'complete' protein as it contains all nine of the essential amino acids. It is gluten free and a good source of calcium. Quinoa is also lower in carbohydrates than rice. A 100 gram portion contains 64 grams whereas the same portion of white rice contains 80.

One thing to remember about quinoa is that it is coated with a toxin called saponin so it is important that you wash it well before cooking it. Rinse the grain in two changes of water. The best way of cooking it is to add two parts water to one part well drained quinoa, bring to the boil and then simmer very slowly for 25 minutes until the water is absorbed. Then leave it to stand for ten minutes. When quinoa is fully cooked the seeds expand and burst open to release a small curly tail.

### Millet

Millet is a gluten free wholegrain that has a sweet nutty flavour. It is considered to be the most digestible and non allergic of the grains. Like Quinoa it is high in protein. As it contains around 15% protein it makes a valuable addition to your diet. Like oatmeal it contains antioxidants and high levels of magnesium. Millet is the staple food of millions of people around the world and like quinoa and oatmeal is has stood the test of time.

Use it in exactly the same way as you would use rice and other grains, hot or cold in salads. Like quinoa it takes a fairly long time to cook and it needs to be cooked using the absorption method, one part millet to two parts water, brought to the boil and then simmered very gently for about half an hour until the water is absorbed. Leave it to stand for ten minutes.

### Bulgar wheat, Spelt and Barley

While all of these grains are mildly inflammatory they still form a valuable part of a gout diet as they are complex carbohydrates and have a low glycemic index. Spelt is particularly interesting as it is an early ancestor of wheat that is more nutritious than wheat and contains less gluten. At 66 grams per 100 grams it also contains less carbohydrate than other wheat type wholegrains.

You can use whole grains of spelt and barley to make risottos as a substitute for rice. Go heavy on the vegetables you add, a risotto does not have to be just rice. Bulgar wheat, spelt and barley make great cold salads when mixed with vegetables and lightly toasted seeds and nuts.

## Cooking Quinoa

*Quinoa is not the easiest of grains to cook as it needs long, very slow cooking. The best way to cook it is by using the absorption method. One part quinoa needs just slightly under two parts of water. The easiest way to do this is to use a small 5fl oz/150 ml dish like a ramekin dish. This holds about 100g/3½ oz of quinoa. Even if the packet says the quinoa is already washed, wash and drain it again.*

*You can cook quinoa on the hob or in the microwave.*

*To cook it on the hob, put the quinoa into a saucepan, bring it to the boil, cover with a tight fitting lid and reduce to a very low heat. Leave it to cook for 25 – 30 minutes. When it has finished cooking leave it to stand for at least a quarter of an hour before taking off the lid.*

*To cook it in the microwave, put the quinoa into a microwave bowl with the water. Cover it loosely and microwave on full power for 10 minutes. Give it a stir, put the cover back on and leave it to stand for 10 minutes. Then microwave it again on full power for 4 minutes and leave it to stand for 3 – 4 minutes before serving.*

*Troublesome it may be to cook, but quinoa is packed full of protein and it has a low glycemic index. Of all of the grains it is probably the healthiest one to eat.*

*To freeze quinoa all you need to do is open freeze it on a large tray lined with cling film or non stick foil and when it is frozen put it into a box or a bag so that you can use it as and when needed. It thaws out very quickly once it is taken out of the freezer.*

## Cooking Millet

*Like most grains the best way to cook millet is by using the absorption method. Like quinoa one part millet needs about two parts of water. The easiest way to do this is to use a small 5fl oz/150 ml ramekin dish. This holds about 100g/3½ oz of millet.*

*To cook it on the hob, put the millet into a saucepan, bring it to the boil, cover with a tight fitting lid and reduce to a very low heat. Leave it to cook for 35 – 40 minutes. When it has finished cooking add a tablespoon of boiling water, put the lid back on and leave it to stand for a quarter of an hour before taking off the lid.*

## Cooking Whole Buckwheat

*Unlike millet and quinoa whole buckwheat is best covered with cold water, brought to the boil and then simmered very gently for between 20 to 25 minutes. Drain before serving.*

## Cooking Pearl Barley & Pearl Spelt

*As with buckwheat these are best covered with cold water, brought to the boil and then simmered slowly. Make sure you wash the spelt or barley well before cooking it as it tends to be quite dusty. Pearl spelt needs to simmer for about 20 minutes but pearl barley will need to simmer for 50 minutes before it is cooked.*

## Cooking Couscous.

*Couscous is made from wheat and sometimes barley. It comes in fine, medium and giant forms. Because it it pre-processed couscous is by far the easiest 'grain' to prepare. All you need to do is add 1 part couscous to 2 parts boiling water, give it a stir and then leave it to stand for 5 – 10 minutes. Medium couscous needs to be gently simmered for 5 minutes before being left to stand. Giant couscous needs to be simmered for 10 minutes.*

## Cooking Bulgar Wheat

*Bulgar wheat is a whole cracked part processed wheat that like couscous comes in fine, medium and course varieties. It is cooked in exactly the same way as couscous.*

*For fine bulgar wheat add 1 part couscous to 2 parts boiling water, give it a stir and then leave it to stand for 5 – 10 minutes. Medium bulgar wheat needs to be gently simmered for 5 minutes before being left to stand. Course bulgar wheat needs to be simmered for 10 minutes.*

## Toasted Oatmeal Coating

*This is a useful mixture of oatmeal, spices and seeds that can be used as a crunchy topping for bakes an gratins and as a coating for burgers.*

SERVES 4

200g/7oz flaked oatmeal

3 tbsp olive oil

3 tbsp water

A handful of sunflower seeds

½ tsp ground turmeric

1 tsp garlic granules

1 tbsp dried oregano

1 tsp chilli flakes

Pre heat the oven to 160°C/ 325°F/Gas 3

1. Grease a 20cm/8 in square baking tin and line the base with baking parchment or non stick foil.
2. Mix the flaked oats and sunflower seeds with the turmeric, garlic granules, chilli flakes and oregano.
3. Put the water and olive oil into a saucepan and bring it to the boil.
4. Add the oil and water for the flaked oats. Mix well and press the mixture into the prepared tin. Bake for 30 minutes until the oats are golden brown.
5. Leave the oats to cool completely, then use a rolling pin to break the oats down into large crumbs.

Store in an airtight tin or freeze.

## Date & Muesli Bars

*Moist chewy biscuits that are quick and easy to make and keep for up to a week in an airtight tin. The mashed banana works wonders as it takes the place of egg and binds the ingredients together.*

---

Makes 9 - 16

2 large ripe bananas
1 heaped tbsp dark unrefined Muscavado sugar
2 tbsp olive oil
120g/4¼ oz chopped dates
30g/1oz pumpkin seeds
3 tsp mixed spice
½ tsp ground ginger
200g/7oz flaked oatmeal
50g/1¾oz chopped pecan nuts or walnuts

---

You will need a 20cm/8 in greased square tin, preferably silicon bakeware. Pre heat the oven to 160°C/ 325°F/Gas 3.

1. Put the bananas into a bowl and use a hand blender to whiz them into a smooth purée. Add the olive oil and blend until mixed.
2. Mix together the flaked oatmeal, muscavado sugar, mixed spice and ground ginger in a separate bowl. If the sugar is lumpy break it up with your fingers.
3. Stir in the nuts, pumpkin seeds and chopped dates.
4. Add the banana and oil to the oatmeal, seeds and nuts and mix thoroughly. The mixture will be fairly dry. Put it into the prepared tin and, using the back of a spoon, press it down firmly.
5. Cook for 30 minutes until the biscuit is firm to the touch and beginning to look slightly golden around the edge. Take it out of the oven and put to one side to cool a little.
6. When it is cool enough to handle put the biscuit onto a chopping board and use a sharp knife to cut it into 9 or16 pieces.

## Pasta & Pizza – in any shape you want

*Pasta and Pizza are to most of us synonymous with 'fast food' and, despite their relatively healthy Mediterranean origins, in the western diet, they have evolved into a notoriously unhealthy food.*

**Why?**

Even though pasta is a carbohydrate food that is made from refined wheat, pasta has a medium to low glycemic index. So like whole grains, it takes longer to digest and metabolise and as a consequence it releases its glucose more slowly. The low to medium glycemic index of pasta appears to come from the stretching and rolling process it goes through when it is made. This entraps some of the starch granules in a sponge like network of protein molecules in the pasta dough. Asian noodles such as Udon and rice vermicelli also have a low to medium GI.

Pasta comes in many different shapes and sizes and it is quick and easy to prepare. It should be cooked al dente or 'firm to bite', in other words it should be slightly firm and offer some resistance when you chew it. This is the best way to eat it as the more it is cooked the higher its glycemic index becomes.

Why is pasta in the 'sort of good' and not 'the good' category?

Two reasons. First, the flour it is made from is fortified with iron and the gout diet aims to reduce the amount of iron you consume. Secondly, it is made from wheat and all wheat products are mildly to moderately inflammatory. So limit the amount you eat and, by combining it with ingredients that are anti-inflammatory, the pro-inflammatory effect can be balanced out; anchovies, sardines, salmon, onion, garlic, chilli, turmeric and spinach are all powerful anti-inflammatory foods.

Interestingly, if you cook pasta until it is 'al dente' and then leave it to cool to room temperature it's glycaemic index reduces further because the starch molecules 'rearrange' themselves during the cooling process and become more resistant to being digested. If you reheat the pasta with a sauce and some vegetables it's glycemic index is reduced even more. So simply by cooking, cooling and reheating pasta you can increase the amount of resistant starch it contains. Provided it is rinsed and cooled quickly after you have cooked it you can keep cooked pasta in a covered container in the fridge for up to 3 days. It also freezes well.

Whole wheat pasta contains less iron and more fibre than pasta made from refined white flour. Because of this when you eat whole wheat pasta you feel fuller for longer. However, if you eat white pasta with plenty of vegetables the fibre in the vegetables will also give you the 'full' feeling. Whether you use whole wheat or white pasta is a matter of personal choice.

To most of us Pizza means bread dough, usually thick but sometimes thin, with some form of topping and cheese. Usually a Pizza is more 'bread' than topping and often more 'cheese' than topping. Commercial Pizza especially, with far too much salt and sugar added, it is not a particularly healthy food, but this is not necessarily the way 'Pizza' is made in Mediterranean countries. There are many different types of 'Pizza' and most of them are loaded with herbs and spices and these go some way to mitigating the inflammatory effect of the wheat. Almost without exception they also have more 'topping' than base.

**How:**

Although most manufacturers specify a cooking time, because over cooking increases its glycemic index, when you cook pasta start testing it 2 to 3 minutes before the recommended time is up. The only thing to be mindful of is the total amount of pasta you eat. A 100 gramme portion of uncooked pasta contains about 70 grams of carbohydrate, so eating too much will increase the glucose load.

A cup of al dente pasta combined with plenty of vegetables and some herbs, especially pesto, can be turned into a substantial healthy adult meal. Adding lemon juice or vinegar and eating it with beans will also reduce its glycemic index by slowing down the rate at which it is digested. Try mixing pasta with pesto, rocket, red beans and semi dried tomatoes, try it combined with cauliflower, capers and anchovies or sardines, garlic and tomato purée and a large bowl of salad. Combined with plenty of vegetables 3 sheets of lasagne makes a meal for two people. Spinach, butter nut squash and walnut is an excellent combination. Instead of cheese sauce on the top use yoghurt or yoghurt mixed with pesto.

## Cauliflower, Tomato & Anchovy Pasta

*This is a quick and easy dish that you can prepare in advance and heat up in the microwave at the last minute. You can use any type of 'large' non spaghetti like pasta to make this. Adjust the amount of garlic and chilli you use to suit your taste. If you add some butter beans or cannellini beans you can make this into a really substantial meal that will feed up to 6 people.*

SERVES 4 - 6

1 large cauliflower
200g/7oz cherry tomatoes cut in half
4 cloves garlic crushed
1 red chilli finely chopped OR 1 tsp Sambol Oelek or chilli paste
50g/1¾oz tin anchovy fillets in olive oil
3 tbsp capers
16 - 20 salted black olives stones removed and cut in half
3 tbsp finely sliced basil
150g/5½oz orchietta, large pasta shells or thick pasta tubes
Crushed black pepper (optional)
400g/14 oz tine butter beans or cannellini beans drained and rinsed
2 tbsp lightly toasted pine nuts
4 tbsp finely grated parmesan or pecorino
2 tbsp olive oil (optional)

1 Cook the pasta in line with the instructions on the packet. Just make sure it is 'al dente' still has some bite when you have finished cooking it. Put it to one side while you make the rest of the dish.

2 Remove the outside leaves from the cauliflower and break the inside into small florets about the size of your thumb. Cook these for about 2 minutes until they are just tender. Drain, reserving about 50ml/2 fl oz of the cooking liquid and put to one side.

3 Drain the oil from the anchovies into a large saucepan or wok and cut the anchovies into 1 cm/½ in pieces.

4 Heat the oil from the anchovies over a medium heat and add the garlic and the chilli. Because of the fluid in it the oil will spit a little. Cook the garlic and chilli for 2 – 3 minutes but do not let it brown.

5 Stir in the capers, the olives and tomatoes and the reserved cooking liquid from the cauliflower. Now stir in the cooked pasta, the cauliflower and, if you are using them, the beans. Cover and cook slowly just long enough to heat through.

6 Just before serving stir in half of the grated parmesan or pecorino and sprinkle on the shredded basil and toasted pine nuts.Serve the rest of the parmesan in separate bowl.

## Courgette & Red Pepper Lasagne

*Ready to use lasagne makes lasagne fairly quick and easy to make. Even though the instructions on the packet do not tell you to, pre-soaking the sheets of lasagne while you prepare the filling improves the texture. You will need a 5cm/2 in deep large ovenproof dish or casserole that takes 3 sheets of lasagne across the base to make this.*

*A dish that is 24cm x 20 cm or 10 in x 8 in is ideal. You will find the recipe for basil pesto on page130.*

SERVES 6

9 sheets ready to use lasagne
6 spring onions finely sliced
1 clove garlic crushed (optional)
400g/14 oz can chopped tomatoes
3 tbsp tomato purée
1 tsp cayenne pepper
4 tbsp fromage frais or natural unsweetened yoghurt
3 large free range eggs
3 tbsp finely grated parmesan.
2 large red peppers
400g/14 oz courgettes thinly sliced

For the topping:
350g/12oz packet silken tofu
100ml/3½ fl oz milk
1 large free range egg
60g/2¼oz basil pesto
3 tbsp finely grated parmesan

1 Pre heat the oven to 200°C/ 400°F/Gas 5 and grease the baking dish.

2 Put the sheets of lasagne into a large shallow bowl and cover them with hot water. Leave them to soak while you prepare the filling.

3 Cut the red peppers into quarters and remove the seeds. Put them onto a baking tray lined with non stick foil and roast them for 20 to 25 minutes. Tip them into a bowl and cover them with cling film.

4 Put the sliced courgette into a microwave bowl, cover and cook for 3 minutes until it is just beginning to soften.

5 Whisk the eggs, tomato purée, cayenne pepper, fromage frais and parmesan together. Stir in the spring onions, the copped tomatoes and the garlic. If there is any fluid in the bowl with the courgettes drain this off and stir this in as well.

6 When the peppers are cool enough to handle remove the cling film and peel off the skin. You do not need to remove all of the skin, but make sure you take off any skin that looks black and charred. Keep any oil that is in the bowl.

7 Drain the sheets of lasagne. Put 3 sheets of the lasagne in a layer on the bottom of the ovenproof dish. Spoon on a third of the tomato mixture. On top of this arrange the courgettes is an even layer and then spoon on another third of the tomato mixture on top.

8 Put 3 sheets of lasagne on top of this and then add the roasted red peppers. Pour on any oil that is in the bowl. Spoon on the last of the tomato mixture and put the last 3 sheets of lasagne on top.

9 Use a hand blender to mix the tofu with the pesto, egg, milk and 2 tablespoons of the grated parmesan. Pour this on top. Cover with foil and bake for 30 minutes at 200°C/ 400°F/Gas 5. Remove the foil and sprinkle on the remaining tablespoon of grated parmesan and cook for another 10 minutes.

## Pasta a Faglio

*This is an adaptation of a classic Italian dish that is more like a stew than a soup. The authentic dish uses dried borlotti beans that are soaked overnight before being cooked. Canned beans are much quicker. You can cook the pasta in advance and add it to the stew at the last minute.*

SERVES 6

2 x 400g/14 ox can of borlotti beans drained and rinsed
1 large onion finely sliced
3 tbsp olive oil
1 large leek finely sliced
2 large carrots peeled and finely chopped
2 sticks celery finely chopped
1 large potato peeled and chopped into 1cm/½ in dice
4 cloves of garlic crushed
600ml/20fl oz (1pt) vegetable stock
½ tsp dried thyme
½ tsp dried rosemary
½ tsp dried sage
200g/7oz conchiglie or small pasta shells
10 large tomatoes each cut into 8 pieces
2 tbsp tomato purée
Salt and ground black pepper
Finely grated parmesan and finely Chopped parsley or chervil to serve

1 Heat the olive oil in a large saucepan and add the sliced onions, leeks, potatoes and carrots. Sauté for 5 minutes and then add the garlic, thyme, rosemary and sage.

2 Stir in the vegetable stock, the tomato purée and the borlotti beans. Bring to the boil, reduce the heat, cover and leave the 'stew' simmering while you cook the pasta.

3 Add the pasta to a large saucepan of boiling water. Cook for 7 to 8 minutes until it is just cooked, then drain it.

4 Add the pasta to the bean stew and stir in the tomatoes. Scatter some chopped parsley and grated parmesan over the top and serve the rest of the parmesan in a separate bowl.

## Pizza with Onions & Anchovies

*Not quite the pizza we are used to but just as good, and it is much quicker to make as there is no need to prove the dough or roll out the base. The pizza 'crust' is an adaptation of an 18th Century recipe for soda bread that was made with oatmeal and wholegrain flour.*

*You can make the pizza base and use any type of topping, with or without tomato and with or without cheese. This recipe uses just onions and olives, a way pizza is often served in Rome. Both the pizza base and the onion confit used as the topping can be made in advance and stored in the fridge. They also freeze well.*

SERVES 4

For the pizza base:
60g/2¼oz wholegrain spelt
60g/2¼oz fine oatmeal
1 tsp baking powder
3 tbsp olive oil
250ml/9 fl oz milk

For the topping:
450g/1lb white onions finely sliced
100g/3½oz soft low fat cheese such as Quark or ricotta
Finely grated zest of ½ lemon
Juice of ½ lemon
2 bay leaves
Crushed black pepper
50g/1¾oz tin anchovy fillets in olive oil
24 salted black olives stones removed and cut in half
2 tbsp pine nuts

1 You will need a 24cm/10 in round silicon tin or spring form tin to make this. If you are using an ordinary tin grease it well.
2 First make the onion confit. Drain half of the oil from the anchovies into a saucepan, add the onions and gently sauté them over a medium heat for 5 minutes.
3 Add the bay leaves and lemon zest, cover the saucepan, reduce the heat to low and simmer the onions for 30 – 40 minutes until they are soft. Check them once in a while to make sure they are not burning, sticking or turning brown. Add a tablespoon of water if you need to.

4 Remove the bay leaves and leave the onions to cool slightly before stirring in the lemon juice and the ricotta.

Pre heat the oven to 200°C/ 400°F/Gas 5

5 To make the pizza base. Mix the spelt, fine oatmeal and baking powder together.

6 Whisk the olive oil into the milk.

7 Add the milk and oil to the flour. It will start bubbling as soon as the milk is added to the flour so mix it quickly to form a batter and pour it into the baking tin. Put it into the oven straight away and bake for 12 minutes. By this time it should be lightly browned and firm to the touch. Turn it over and put it back into the oven for 3 minutes to dry off the base.

8 To assemble the pizza, put the pizza base onto an ovenproof plate or baking tray and spoon on the onion mixture. Arrange the black olives and anchovies on top and sprinkle on the pine nuts. Drizzle over the remaining oil from the anchovy fillets. Bake for 10 minutes to heat the topping through.

## Cheats Calzone with Refried Beans

*If you want a really quick meal every so often you can make this with commercial tortillas from the Supermarket and a commercial sweet chilli sauce. Yes, the commercial sweet chilli sauce will probably contain mono sodium glutamate as well as sugar but it's what you do most of the time not what you do some of the time that matters. You can use any type of hard cheese, goats or sheep's cheese is very good. Serve the calzone with refried beans and some salad.*

*You can serve refried beans on their own or as an accompaniment to tortillas and frittatas as well as with the cheats calzone.*

---

Makes 4 small calzone
4 commercial tortillas
4 tbsp sweet chilli sauce
2 ripe avocados
2 tbsp lemon or lime juice
8 tbsp grated cheese

For the refired beans
400g/14 oz can red or black beans drained and rinsed
1 medium white onion finely sliced
2 tbsp olive oil
2 cloves garlic crushed
1 tsp chilli powder
½ tsp smoked paprika1 tsp ground cumin
Finely grated zest and juice of a lime
150ml/5 fl oz (¼ pt) water
2 tbsp chopped coriander

---

1. To make the refried beans. Heat the oil in a saucepan, add the sliced onion and sauté for 5 minutes. Stir in the crushed garlic, chilli power, smoked paprika and ground cumin.
2. Sauté for 2 to 3 minutes, then add the beans, lime zest and the water. Bring to the boil, cover, reduce the heat and simmer for 15 minutes.
3. Just before serving stir in the lime juice and blend briefly with a hand blender to break down some of the beans.
4. To make the calzone. Pre heat the oven to 180°C/ 350°F/Gas 4.

5. Cut the avocados in half and use a small spoon to remove the stone. Peel the avocados and slice them thinly. Drizzle the lemon juice over them to prevent them turning brown.
6. Microwave the tortillas for 30 seconds to make them pliable.
7. Put the tortillas onto a board. Spread a tablespoon of the sweet chilli sauce over one half. Put the slices of one half of an avocado on top and sprinkle on 2 tablespoon of grated cheese Fold the tortilla over to cover the filling.
8. Put the calzone onto a baking tray lined with non stick foil and bake for 10 minutes.

## Rice

*- in the form of basmati rice, risotto rice, brown rice and rice noodles. but not long grain rice, Thai Jasmine rice and 'easy cook' rice.*

**Why?**

Rice is the staple food of millions of people around the world and it is cheap and easy to cook. However, it contains large amounts of glycemic starch, a starch that is a converted into sugar and absorbed almost as quickly as the sugar in a soft drink. One hundred grams of uncooked white rice contains about 80 grams of carbohydrate, around 7 grams of protein and only 1.3 grams of dietary fibre and it is the small amount of fibre that is the problem with white rice. As most of the fibre, vitamins and minerals in rice are in the layer of husk and bran that is removed when the rice is polished, it is not surprising that brown rice is far more nutritious than white rice.

Eating boiled rice as a staple food is something of a paradox. We are told to be careful about how much rice we eat as it *'makes us fat'* and yet Asians, Chinese and Japanese eat it two or three times a day and as a general rule they stay slim. How and why this happens is unclear but what is clear is that scientists have now discovered a way of improving the nutritional content of rice by cooking it in a different way. Simply by adding a small amount of butter, olive oil or coconut oil to the water the rice is cooked in and then cooking the rice, cooling it quickly and leaving it in the fridge for 12 to 24 hours, some of the glycemic starch in the rice is changed into resistant starch, a fibre that we digest slowly. Contrary to what you would expect, reheating the rice when you are ready to eat it increases the amount of resistant starch even more.

*Should you worry about the arsenic in rice?*

As well as being toxic arsenic is also a major carcinogen. Just about all soil and water contains arsenic and small amounts find their way into our food. Usually there is not enough arsenic to worry about but because rice is grown in water it contains between ten and twenty times more arsenic than other cereals. The World Health Organisation and the EU have both set guidelines for the amount of arsenic that is permitted, both in rice itself and products that are made from rice.

As with vitamins, minerals and fibre the husk and bran of rice contains a lot of the arsenic so brown rice contains more than white rice. For most of us if we eat rice in moderation as part of a balanced diet the amount of arsenic we consume should not be a problem. There is however, something you can do about it and, as with fibre, it is all to do with the way the rice is cooked. Even if you rinse it first, cooking rice by the absorption method means that all of the arsenic stays in the rice. If you boil the rice in plenty of water and then rinse it, about half of the arsenic is removed. However, if you soak the rice overnight and then rinse it before boiling it in plenty of water between 70% and 80% of the arsenic will be removed. So if you add some fat or oil to the cooking water and then rinse the rice in cold water before keeping it in the fridge, you remove most of the arsenic, increase the amount of resistant starch the rice contains and transform it into a much healthier food.

### How

Instead of being quick and easy to cook soaking, boiling and rinsing makes cooking rice a bit of a chore, but provided the rice is cooled quickly, cooked rice can be safely kept for up to two days in a covered container in the fridge. But the good news is that rice freezes really well and you can use it straight from the freezer.

Unlike other rice, basmati rice and brown rice have a low to medium glycemic index. Brown rice has a GI of 48 and basmati rice has a GI of 57. The GI of other rice and 'easy cook' rice is much higher. For instance Thai jasmine rice has a GI of 89. As with all carbohydrates the more the rice is cooked the higher its glycemic index becomes so try not to overcook it. Cooking times vary but a high quality white basmati rice will be cooked in about 10 minutes. The cooking times for brown rice are much longer.

As with pasta you need to be mindful that rice is high in carbohydrates. Try making it into a pilaf by combining it with vegetables, lemon juice and beans. As well as reducing its GI still further this transforms a modest amount of rice into a substantial meal. Rice, carrots, chick peas, cumin and coriander is a classical Indian pilaf. Yoghurt and mint makes a great addition as a side dish.

## Broad Bean & Almond Pilaf

*This can be cooked in advance and reheated when you are ready to serve it. You can also use quinoa, basmati rice, pearl barley, spelt or buckwheat to make this.*

SERVES 4

200g/7oz basmati rice cooked, rinsed and cooled
300g/10½oz frozen broad beans
2 tbsp olive oil
3 medium white onions finely sliced
3 cloves garlic crushed
1 tsp vegetable stock powder
1 tsp cayenne pepper
1 tbsp cumin seeds
3 tbsp raisins
40g/1½ oz flaked almonds
2 tbsp lemon juice
Salt and pepper to taste

Pre heat the oven to 180°C/ 350°F/Gas 4

1 Put the almonds onto a baking try and cook them for 7 to 8 minutes until they are light golden brown.
2 Sauté the onions in the oil over a medium heat for 5 minutes. Add the garlic, cayenne pepper and cumin seeds and cook for 2 – 3 minutes.
3 Add 4 tablespoons of water, the vegetable stock powder and the raisins. Bring to the boil, cover, reduce the heat to very low and cook slowly for 2 minutes.
4 Stir in the rice and turn off the heat. Put the rice and onions into a microwave bowl, cover and cook on full power for 5 minutes while you cook the broad beans.
5 Bring the broad beans to the boil and cook for 6 - 7 minutes. Drain and, if you are inclined to or believe you should, peel them.
6 Add the broad beans to the rice and raisins and stir in the lemon juice. Sprinkle the toasted almonds on top and serve.

## The Humble Potato

**Why?**

Despite having a very high glycemic index, cooked the right way potatoes come into the 'sort of good' as opposed to 'bad' category.

**How?**

Baking them is not a good idea as, depending of the variety, the glycemic index of a medium size baked potato can be between 85 and 95. However, there are other ways of cooking them that can reduce this figure significantly. For example lightly sautéing potatoes in olive oil versus boiling them will lower their glycemic index because it adds fat and is less destructive to the starchy potato carbohydrate. Just remember that olive oil is a high energy food so use it in moderation. Steaming potatoes results in a lower glycemic index than boiling or microwaving. Leaving the skin on a potato as opposed to peeling it will retain some of the insoluble fibre as well as vitamins and minerals. The fibre will slow down its digestion and lower the impact of the starch in the potato on blood glucose levels and as a consequence reduce its glycemic index.

Potato salad made the day before and dressed with lemon, vinegar or vinaigrette is another good way of preparing them. As with rice, keeping cooked potatoes in the fridge overnight leaves them with a much lower GI as opposed to eating them as soon as they are cooked. Keeping cooked potatoes in the cold can reduce their starch content by as much as one third and the acid in the vinaigrette, irrespective of whether you use lemon juice, lime juice or vinegar will slow down the rate at which they are digested and metabolised.

Cold potatoes, chopped dill cucumbers, chopped walnuts and fresh dill makes a particularly tasty salad. Add a few chopped cured herrings and you have a meal.

## Nordic Salad

*A classic way of serving oily fish like herrings, mackerel and sardines that have been preserved. This recipe uses cold potatoes but you could use cannellini beans as an alternative.*

---

SERVES 4

Large 500g/1lb 2oz jar Bismark Herring or Roll mops
1 small red onion finely sliced
700g/1 lb 9oz cooked waxy salad potatoes
100g/3½ oz small pickled gherkins
250g/9oz cooked sweetcorn kernels
Hand full of parsley, chervil or dill finely chopped

Baby salad leaves to serve

---

1 Either slice the cooked potatoes or cut them into 1cm/½ in dice.
2 Slice the gherkins into thin rounds.
3 Wash and drain the sweetcorn.
4 Put the potatoes and gherkins into a large serving dish and add the sweetcorn kernels and the sliced onion.
5 Cut the Bismark Herrings or Roll mops into bite size pieces and place them on top.
6 Garnish with the chopped herbs and serve on a bed of baby salad leaves.

## Salmon With Cucumber & Potato Salsa

*You can use salmon or trout for this recipe. The fish can be served hot or cold, either as a fillet or broken into bite size pieces. The cucumber and potato salsa will keep in the fridge for 2 days.*

---

SERVES 4

4 fillets of salmon each weighing about 150g/5½oz
½ lemon thinly sliced
4 bay leaves.
For the Salsa:
16 - 20 small cooked new potatoes
1 large telegraph cucumber, peeled, cut in half lengthways and de-seeded
8 spring onions finely chopped
1 finely chopped green chilli
1 - 2 cloves of garlic crushed
2 tbsp capers drained and roughly chopped
1 tbsp finely chopped fresh dill
1 tbsp chopped flat leaf parsley or chervil
Finely grated zest of 2 limes
Juice of 2 limes
2 tbsp olive oil
Sprigs of fresh dill or parsley to garnish.

---

Pre heat the oven to 200°C/ 400°F/Gas 5

1 Line a small baking try with foil. Put the fillets of salmon on the foil, skin side down and tuck a bay leaf under each one. Arrange the slices of lemon on top of the fish and cover with a piece of foil. Turn over all 4 edges to seal the fish in a large parcel.

2 Bake the fish for 20 minutes until it is set and translucent. The precise time it takes will depend on the thickness of the fish. When the fish is cooked take it out of the oven but leave it in the foil to rest while you prepare the salsa.

3 Cut the potatoes and cucumber into small 5mm/¼ in dice and put them into a large bowl. Add the spring onions, chilli, garlic, capers, dill, parsley and lime zest and give everything a good stir.

4 Put the lime juice and olive oil into a small jar, put on the lid and give it a good shake. Mix this into the potato and cucumber.

5 When you are ready to serve the fish, put a small pile of the salsa onto a plate and place the fillet of fish on top. Garnish with the herbs.

## Coffee

*Coffee is another paradox when it comes to hyperuricemia and gout. Put simply, if you are already drinking a moderate amount of coffee every day then its fine. But if you do not drink coffee on a regular basis it is not a good idea to start.*

**Why:**

Studies have shown that coffee is associated with reduced levels of uric acid and a lower risk of type two diabetes. The caffeine in coffee is a Xanthine, trimethyl-xanthine, and this is thought to exert a protective effect against gout in a way that is similar to the way Allopurinol works through Xanthine Oxidase inhibition. However, all coffee contains caffeine and caffeine tends to promote the breakdown and excretion of calcium salts. So drinking a lot, four or more cups a day, may increase the amount of calcium ions and these can potentially contribute to the seeding of monosodium urate crystals.

The bottom line is the intermittent use of coffee or the sudden introduction of a large amount of coffee could potentially trigger an attack of gout, in much the same way as the therapeutic introduction of Allopurinol can.

# The Bad

## Carbohydrates:

*When consumed in excess all types of carbohydrates are bad, irrespective of whether it is the starch found in bread, rice and potatoes or sugar in all its forms and disguises. And remember, alcohol (ethanol) is metabolised in exactly the same way as fructose, so alcohol effectively counts as carbohydrates.*

### Why?

It is thought that primitive man consumed around 80 gram of carbohydrate a day. Today, on average, we are consuming between 350 and 600 grams. A massive increase and our bodies are just not designed to cope with it. If you have gout you will almost certainly also have hyperuricemia as cases of gout without hyperuricemia are rare. It also means that you will either be insulin resistant or near to becoming insulin resistant. This affects your body's ability to excrete uric acid and it also leads to a state of chronic inflammation and an environment in which the oxidation of fats and lipid peroxidation can take place at an alarming rate.

### How?

As an initial step, try to reduce your consumption of carbohydrates to between 50 and 100 grams a day. This sounds a bit extreme but it is the first step on the road to recovery. You need to regulate your insulin, get it under control and reset your insulin sensitivity. Once your insulin sensitivity is under control you will be able to relax a bit and increase the amount of carbohydrate you eat to between 100 and 150 grams a day.

This is easier said than done as many foods contain 'hidden' carbohydrates. When we think about carbohydrates we automatically think of bread, rice, pasta, potatoes and cakes. But remember, fruit and vegetables also contain carbohydrates in the form of starch and sugar. Banana is a great food that you should most definitely be eating. Just remember that it is quite high in carbohydrates and these carbohydrates are in the form of sugar. Know how much you are eating, so as you start the diet, weigh the banana and other fruit.

Stop eating packaged and processed foods. Most of us eat them every day. They are loaded with carbohydrates and sugar and have little to no nutritional value. Switch to complex whole grain carbohydrates and foods made from them, whether cracked, crushed or rolled. They contain the essential parts and nutrients of the entire grain or seed and these are needed to build your body's antioxidant defence team. Change from white and wholemeal bread to whole grain bread, pumpernickel type rye or spelt. Better still, have a go at making your own bread using spelt and rye flour. It doesn't have to be yeast bread either. Soda bread is great and it only takes minutes to prepare. But take care. Bread contains a lot of carbohydrate.

Use cooking methods that reduce the glycemic index of the carbohydrate foods you eat and try mixing them with foods that are high in fibre as this slows down the rate at which they are absorbed and converted into glucose.

**Tips:**

We live in a culture that expects to have a portion of carbohydrates with each meal and moving away from this takes some doing. Try substituting lightly cooked mashed cauliflower for rice. Shredded cabbage 'tagliatelle' works well. Beans like borlotti, fava beans, chickpeas and butter beans are a great source of protein and fibre as well as carbohydrate and they contain far less carbohydrate than the same weight of potatoes, rice or pasta.

## Sugar and High Fructose Corn Syrup

**Why:**

Because your body simply does not need sugar, irrespective of what form it comes in. It can make all the glucose it needs from the carbohydrates you consume, even when you have reduced your carbohydrate intake. All consuming sugar and fructose will do is increase your insulin sensitivity, increase the amount of uric acid you are producing and reduce the amount of uric acid you are excreting. It will also contribute to a few extra pounds in body weight.

**How:**

Its easier said than done especially if you eat a lot of convenience foods and you drink a lot of non diet carbonated soft drinks. You can cut sugar out of drinks like tea and coffee by using an artificial sweetener. Stevia is the current favourite, but better still, try to retrain your palette. It is not easy but there are some very helpful web sites that can help.

The difficult part about cutting out sugar and High Fructose Corn Syrup is that so many foods contain them; ice cream, mayonnaise and salad dressings are loaded with them as well as trans fats and even 'ready meals' and TV diners have them added as browning agents. In fact they are used in just about all processed foods as a preservative and 'regular' non diet soft drinks and squashes contain an enormous amount, up to 10 teaspoons of sugar (40 grams !) in a 12 oz or 350cc drink.

There is no easy solution to cutting out sugar and HFCS. You are either going to have to stop consuming these types of food completely or start making your own, without sugar.

**Tips:**

- Avoid fast foods.
- Substitute fizzy water for carbonated soft drinks. Ignore the stuff on the internet that says carbonated fizzy water is bad for you. It is yet more misinformation. Ten teaspoons of sugar in each can of soft drink damages your health far more than carbonated water.

- Make your own lemonade. It freezes really well and the Vitamin C is not damaged by freezing.
- Green, white and oolong teas are great and they are really good for you. In fact they form an essential part of a good gout diet.
- Read the labels on food very carefully and beware of the word 'natural'. Remember fructose is a natural sugar!
- Be wary of anything in a box or packet with a long shelf life. Sugar and fructose is often used as a preservative.

## Polyunsaturated Vegetable Oils and Trans Fats

*Sunflower, safflower, rapeseed, canola, peanut (ground nut or arachide) and soya oils as well as margarines and spreads.*

### Why?

Because they are major sources of highly reactive free radicals that have the potential to severely damage your health. They also contribute to a major imbalance between the Omega 3 and Omega 6 essential fatty acids and this makes them highly inflammatory. In fact the amount of Omega 6 in a typical Western Diet can make inflammation run out of control. Hot pressed polyunsaturated vegetable oils are totally man made products and they are most definitely not good for you.

How many convenience foods do you consume in a day?

A typical Western diet has about 30% of its calories from polyunsaturated vegetable oils. These are incorporated into cell membranes where they wreak havoc, disrupting cell metabolism and ultimately damaging or killing the cell. When this happens free radicals and uric acid are released into the blood stream, resulting in increased pressure on your antioxidant defences and oxidative stress.

### How?

Switch to butter and olive oil. They are healthy foods that have both stood the test of time. Goose fat and lard are also alternatives but take care and use all of these in moderation. Fat is a high energy food so it contains a lot of calories; just 8 grams of butter contains 50 kcal and 1 tablespoon olive oil contains 120 kcal. If you want to use salad dressings make your own; flax and hemp seed oils are good as well as olive oil. When you buy any oil make sure you read the label carefully and buy only oils that have been 'cold pressed'. Oil that is in a dark bottle is best as it protects the oil from sunlight and also keep the oil in the fridge as this also reduces the rate at which it oxidises.

A note about labelling legislation as this varies enormously between countries. In the EU cold pressed means just that, but in many other countries labels are simply marketing tools that can say more or less anything.

*Which foods contain polyunsaturated oils and trans fats?*

In terms of trans fats we are back to the old chestnut of biscuits, cookies, cakes, more or less anything that is processed, as well as margarines, 'spreadable' butter, non dairy creamers. The number of products containing polyunsaturated vegetable oils is enormous; crisps, chips, fries, salad dressings, mayonnaise, anything that is fried commercially. It really is staggering how these unhealthy oils have stealthily found their way into our food and even more staggering how they are so often presented as 'the healthy' option.

**Tip:**

A word about rancid and oxidised fat. All fats oxidise and become rancid when they are exposed to heat, light and air and this includes the fat and oils that are in and on meat and fish. Remember the smell and taste of oily fish like sardines when they are a bit old? Because it is 'hung' for sometimes up to ten days in order to tenderise it, meat like beef can contain a lot of rancid oxidised fat. This usually appears yellow. When you cook the meat this fat becomes even more oxidised and rancid. So if you are trying to reduce your consumption of oxidised fat and oil go for freshly slaughtered meat and buy leaner cuts of meat with less fat.

## Alcohol: Beer, Lager, Cider, Wine and Spirits

### Why:

If you suffer from gout you really do need to stop drinking alcohol in order to 'kick start' your return to health. Ethanol in any shape or form simply causes too much damage, and just like fructose, it metabolises very quickly into fat. Not a good idea when we are trying to lose some weight.

Until you get things under control beer and lager are absolute no-no's. I can hear your saying, but years ago people used to drink a lot of beer? Yes they did, but their diet was totally different to ours; small amounts of complex carbohydrates, little or no sugar, only a small amount of meat and loads and loads of vegetables. Interestingly, in the 1800's in London oysters, which are high in Omega-3 essential fatty acids and zinc, were given away free with beer. A much healthier option than a bag of crisps or fries!

### How:

If you regularly drink beer or lager this is going to be very difficult. Alcohol is not an easy habit to break. In adopting this new eating and lifestyle plan you are going to make a lot of changes and some of these will to you be 'sacrifices'. Just keep saying to yourself that each day without a beer brings you one day nearer to leading a gout free life, and that gout free life could well mean a beer when ever you want one.

### Tips:

A switch to red wine would be good as there is no direct link between drinking red wine and gout. But remember, it still contains alcohol and it still contains calories. If you can manage to get through a week of not eating the things you love and feel deprived, you can maybe reward yourself with a piece of 90% chocolate or a small glass of red wine.

## Foods That Contain Iron:

### Why?

If you have gout the amount of iron in your blood is probably quite high. If you have been consuming a typical western diet it is unlikely to be low. High levels of iron are bad for several reasons. Iron is needed to make Xanthine Oxidase, the last enzyme in the process of breaking down and converting purines into uric acid. The more Xanthine Oxidase you have the more uric acid your body is able to make. In addition, iron binds to Vitamin C and destroys its ability to function as an antioxidant. As Vitamin C is something the body tries hard to hang on to, in order to protect the Vitamin C it produces uric acid as this binds to the iron instead. Something of a vicious circle which means that high levels of iron are implicated in stimulating the production of uric acid in two ways.

Over the years high levels of stored iron slowly damage the pancreas and this affects its ability to produce insulin. This ultimately leads to insulin resistance and diabetes, both of which are known to raise levels of uric acid by reducing the amount uric acid that is excreted. Also, when the body is in a state of iron overload the iron can lead to the production of hydroxyl and peroxyl radicals, some of the most highly reactive and dangerous free radicals that can damage cell membranes and give rise to extreme oxidative stress.

### How?

Short of donating blood your body is unable to remove excess iron so you need to reduce your consumption of the foods that contain large amounts of iron; red meat and to a lesser extent poultry. The largest amounts of HEME iron, the iron that is most easily adsorbed and less well regulated by the body comes from red meat. So if you really do want to get on the road to recovery you are going to have to stop eating red meat for a while. If you are eating more vegetables and have cut out alcohol and sugar then your body will not be absorbing as much iron as it was before, but you do need to reduce the overall amount of iron you consume. If you feel unable to cut out meat or animal products completely change from red meat to poultry and fish. They both contain iron but in much smaller amounts. But remember, many manufactured foods are fortified with iron. For example flour, breakfast cereals, breads, pasta as well as any vitamin supplements you may be taking all contain added iron. Alternative sources of protein? Well dare I suggest beans, pulses and tofu. They are excellent sources of protein and the diet of many people in this world is based on them. Tofu and other soy products like tempeh are particularly rich in micro nutrients and some of these micro nutrients like isoflavones are thought to have powerful anti-inflammatory properties.

Remember the Maori? They lived on a diet of fish, poultry and eggs and they lived a gout free life. Once their lifestyle changed and they started eating red meat in large amounts their health deteriorated rapidly.

## Cooking Methods: Frying, Grilling and Roasting

*One of the most intriguing aspects of our modern diet is the high heat at which so much of our food is cooked. None of the food we eat is designed to withstand cooking at such high temperatures. We appear to be addicted to browned, crisp and caramelised food.*

**Why?**

Frying food at high temperatures, especially in polyunsaturated vegetable oils produces large amounts of free radicals. But even without oil, cooking at high temperatures produces some highly damaging substances, such as Advanced Glycation End products or glycotoxins. These are known to be one of the primary factors in degenerative disease and premature ageing. Even in non diabetic men high levels of AGE's reduce levels of testosterone and low levels of testosterone are known to increase the production of uric acid. Not only do AGE's give rise to inflammation, they also damage cells and increase oxidative stress. They are also associated with insulin resistance, diabetes and impaired kidney function, all of which have an impact on both the generation of uric acid and its excretion.

AGE's are created when sugars interact with proteins. Our body's make their own AGE's; the higher the blood sugar level the more AGE's we make and this explains why they have been known about by people studying diabetes for many years. AGE's also come from food and around 10% of the AGE's in our food are absorbed. As only about 3% of these are excreted, over time the levels of AGE's slowly build up.

**How?**

Different foods produce different amounts of AGE's and different cooking methods also give rise to different amounts. Frying, grilling and roasting create the most, whereas boiling, steaming and braising the least. High protein meats, poultry and fish create more than vegetables although chips and fries also contain them.

How many AGE's are we consuming? It is thought that the standard American diet contains three times the recommended safety limit each day. The more raw foods we eat the less AGE's we consume. Interestingly, adding lemon juice or vinegar reduces the number of AGE's that form so marinading food before it is cooked is a good idea. Changing our cooking methods and eating less animal protein will reduce the amount of AGE's our bodies are exposed to. But take care, manufactured foods all contain them, even seemingly innocuous things like flaked breakfast cereals, soy sauce, flavourings and dressings.

Remember the Maori way of cooking? They steamed, boiled and braised their food. Their problems began when they started using an oven and a frying pan.

## Fruit Juice and Smoothies

*The commercial ones that you buy in the Supermarket.*

### Why?

Because they contain enormous amounts of both fructose and glucose as well as preservatives, flavouring and colouring agents. They are not a healthy way to start your day and they are most certainly not one of your 5 a day.

### How?

Eat whole fruit instead of fruit juice, apples, oranges, cranberries, anything the fruit juice is made from. You will be getting the full benefit of the fruit as well as the fibre. There is an old saying that if you are not hungry enough to eat an apple then you are not hungry. You will get far more satisfaction from the 'crunch factor' of one apple than drinking a glass of apple juice that contains the fructose equivalent of three or four.

In terms of smoothies, make your own using fruit and natural unsweetened yoghurt and use the whole fruit whenever possible. If necessary, buy a small blender. Smoothies freeze really well so make them in large quantities. Just take them out of the freezer and leave them to thaw out overnight in the fridge.

## The New Gout Diet: Summary

- Avoid packaged foods, especially those with a long list of ingredients.
- When preparing food select raw, fresh, steamed or boiled foods and avoid fried, BBQ'd, roasted and highly processed foods.

Eat more:-

- Colourful vegetables and fruit; deep red, yellow, orange, green. Eat the rainbow we have all been told to eat. It provides the vitamins, minerals, phytonutrients, fibre and antioxidants that will minimise inflammation. Eat all of these as close as possible to their natural unrefined state as this preserves their beneficial nutrients.
- Healthy fats. Include Omega 3 oils in oily fish, salmon, herring, mackerel, sardines, avocados, olive oil and nuts and seeds in their natural form. And don't be afraid of butter.
- Fibre is one thing many of us have a shortage of in our diet. Yes, it can create flatulence and it also promotes bowel movements but in doing this it creates a favourable environment for healthy bacteria to live in.
- Herbs and spices; parsley, chervil, basil, coriander, garlic, ginger, turmeric. It is a long list. They all contain antioxidants and anti-inflammatory components. The amount they contain is small but every little helps make up a healthy diet.

Eliminate:

- Refined polyunsaturated vegetable oils. Any potential health giving properties have been removed during processing and they are overloaded with Omega 6 fats that fuel inflammation.
- Trans Fats and hydrogenated fats. Our bodies have no means of using them and they are a major source of free radicals and inflammation. Together with polyunsaturated vegetable oils they are the single most damaging food in our modern Western Diet.
- Meat and foods like white flour and breakfast cereals that are enriched with iron. Red meat in particular needs to be eliminated, a least in the short term and if you do eat it make sure it is organically reared grass fed meat.

- High glycemic index and highly processed carbohydrates; bread, pastries, cakes, biscuits, fruit juice are all rapidly digested and lead to rapid rises in blood glucose levels that create insulin spikes and a subsequence inflammatory cascade.
- Artificial sweeteners and preservatives. They have no nutritional value and they promote inflammation.

Make sure that you are not fuelling inflammation with common food allergies or food intolerances; milk, eggs, gluten and peanuts are some of the potential suspects.

We've looked at the 'good', the 'sort of good' and the 'bad' foods. There is no doubt that breaking the eating habits of a lifetime will not be an easy task, but by following these recommendations you will gradually restore your body's natural balance and put yourself on the road to recovery and living a gout free life.

Finally some thoughts to help you on your way.

CHAPTER 11

# Some thoughts to help you on your way

**- Be suspicious about food that is advertised on TV.**

*Most advertising is for processed foods and most of these have additives in the form of sugar or high Fructose Corn Syrup, hydrogenated trans fats, salt and many also have added iron. Food manufacturers spend a lot of money on advertising and look for big returns on their products. This means big profits. They are always one step ahead of the game, so if you buy food that is advertised it will rarely be good for you.*

**- Eat when you are hungry - not because you are bored.**

*Ask yourself why you are eating and whether you are really hungry. If you're not hungry enough to eat an apple you are not hungry.*

**- Understand the difference between thirst and hunger.**

**- Have a drink of water before you reach for something to eat. Better still, make some tea.**

**- Do all of your eating at a table.**

*Don't eat while you are working at a desk, walking around or watching TV. Why? Because when we do this we eat mindlessly and therefore eat more. If you do eat when you are not sitting at the table, eat fruit, vegetables and a few nuts, not chips, crisps, biscuits and burgers.*

**- Reduce the size of your plate !!**

**- Stop eating BEFORE you feel full.**

*Many long lived people in the world stop eating when they are about 80% full.*

**- Don't go to the supermarket to do your shopping when you are hungry.**

*If you do you are more likely to buy fast food, junk food and convenience foods.*

**- Real food does not come in packets and boxes and it does not need a nutritional label.**

**- Carry a magnifying glass with you when you go shopping.**

*If you do need to read labels remember that they are part of the marketing process. The ingredients listed on labels are there to comply with the law, they are not there to provide you with information. Ingredients are always difficult to read as they are invariably in very small print.*

**- If you do buy packaged foods read the label carefully.**

*Contents are often disguised. Maltose and dextrose are still sugar, maltodextrin is still starch and 'enriched' ' usually means that most of the good things have been taken out and a few 'not so good' things put back in. Real food does not need to be 'enriched'.*

**- Cook from scratch as often as you can.**

*There are hidden additives, hydrogenated trans fats and sugars in almost all of the processed and ready-to-eat foods that we don't normally think contain them. Even canned tomatoes can sometimes contain high fructose corn syrup or added sugar, so always check the label.*

**- Convenience foods.**

*It's impossible to break the habits of a lifetime so eat all the convenience foods you want provided you make them yourself. There's nothing wrong with eating fried foods, pastries and ice cream once in a while but manufacturers have made it easy and cheap for us to eat them every day. If you have to make them yourself you will eat them far less often, you certainly won't eat them every day.*

**- If you can buy something for less than the cost of making it yourself there is a reason.**

*Packaged, processed and convenience foods disguise cheap, low quality ingredients, things that you simply should not be eating.*

**- Eating is a social activity.**

*Try not to eat alone. The more you interact with your fellow diners the less you will eat.*

**- Learn to cook. It can be an exciting adventure that gives you a lot of pleasure**

CHAPTER 12

# Conclusion - Is Gout A Wakeup Call?

Gout has afflicted man for thousands of years. It is one of the most painful and debilitating diseases and it affects millions of people around the world. It leaves them facing a lifetime of pain.

If you have ever asked the question "*Why do I have gout*"? you will almost invariably have been told that its because you have too much uric acid, something which is bound to be your fault as it is caused by eating too much purine rich food and drinking too much alcohol. The solution, drugs to reduce the amount of uric acid and a low purine diet. Notwithstanding that a rigid purine restricted diet is well nigh impossible to sustain for long, it a diet that is high in refined carbohydrates and low in the Omega-3 essential fatty acids that your body desperately needs. This will simply make things worse.

Nature has given us some simple and straightforward ways of keeping ourselves healthy. For years we have been told that as uric acid serves no biological purpose our bodies do not need it. Absolutely not true. Uric acid is an important antioxidant and it is also a marker of tissue injury that acts as one of the regulators of our immune system. Uric acid helps our bodies deal with trauma. So when our body is under assault and confronted by an imbalance of free radicals and damaged cells, irrespective of where these come from, our body's antioxidant defences and immune system swing into action in order to put things right. Uric acid levels increase and oxidative stress develops. High levels of uric acid are a warning sign that things are going wrong. They are a sign that our body is out of balance and under stress and that it is calling out for help.

We need a major re-think of how we look at high levels of uric acid and gout. Uric acid is not the bad guy it is made out to be. Rather than using drugs to get rid of the uric acid, a more holistic approach is to find out what is causing the stress and trauma our body is being subjected to and then eliminate the problems. That way we have a chance of getting the body back in balance and functioning normally.

Goodbye To Gout is all about understanding the reasons why we have gout and what we need to do to get our body back into working order. Remember, my husband was crippled by gout. Today he lives a gout free life. I sincerely hope that this book has given you the knowledge and motivation you need to take control of your health and take the first steps towards living a gout free life.

Wishing you all the best.

**Rose Scott**

A Gout Wife

# Appendix

## Sugar

Man's love affair with sugar goes back a long way and it plays an insidious role in our health, especially as in large quantities it is actually quite toxic. For some reason we are in a way almost 'wired' to seek it out, but if sugar is bad for us why do we crave it? The short answer is that like other 'tasty foods' sugar stimulates the same centres in our brain that respond to heroin and cocaine and just like these drugs it has a very pronounced effect. In reality sugar acts on our brain almost like an addictive drug.

Why this happens is interesting as it comes from a time in our evolutionary past when as a result of climate change sugar, in the form of fruit, was only available for a short time of the year. Millions of years ago our early ancestors lived in a tropical climate and were able to eat fruit containing sugar throughout the year. As they moved into Eurasia and the climate cooled the forests became deciduous and fruit was only available for a short time of the year. This resulted in hungry near starving apes and a species that was in decline. At some point a mutation occurred and this made some of the apes extremely efficient at processing the fructose that was found in the seasonal fruit. Even small amounts could be metabolised and very quickly stored as fat. This gave these apes a huge survival advantage. They ate a lot of fruit while they could, put on fat and used the fat to help them survive when food was scarce.

Today all apes, including humans, have this mutation. Our bodies have evolved to survive on very little sugar. So when sugar, especially in its refined form, is available we get fat because we seek it out and we eat far too much of it.

In reality sugar is one of the first 'manufactured' foods. It was first domesticated on the island of New Guinea about 10,000 years ago. The raw sugar cane was chewed and it is thought that the juice extracted from the cane was used in religious ceremonies. Sugar spread slowly from island to island reaching mainland Asia around 1,000BC. By 500AD it had reached India where it was used as a medicine. By 600AD it had spread to Persia and when the Arab armies conquered Persia they took a love of sugar and the knowledge of how to make it back to the Middle East. As the Arab Empire grew, wherever they went sugar went with them and they more or less turned sugar refining into an industry.

Probably the first Europeans to come across sugar were the Crusaders and the first sugar began reaching Europe in small amounts. It was regarded as a spice. It was expensive and only consumed by the wealthy. Some enterprising Crusaders saw an opportunity and began farming and processing sugar cane in small quantities in Cyprus but as the Crusades came to an end the supplies from the Arabs diminished new sources of supply were needed. The hunt was on to find places where sugar cane could be grown and it soon found its way via the Canary and Cape Verde Islands to the Caribbean. As more sugar cane was planted and refined the price of sugar fell and as the price fell so consumption and demand increased. The rest, as they say, is history.

In 1700 the average Englishman consumed 4 pounds of sugar a year. By 1800 he was eating 18 pounds a year and by 1870 consumption had risen to 47 pounds. By 1900 we were consuming 100 pounds a year. Today, about 25 percent of people on a typical 'Western Diet' consume around 95 kilograms or getting on for 200 pounds of sugar a year and for most of us this is more than our body weight. Sounds impossible? Well not when you consider that a 12 ounce can of 'regular' soft drink can contain up to 10 teaspoons of sugar, in others words about 40 grams.

## So what exactly is sugar?

First and foremost sugar is a natural food. It only becomes unnatural when it is in a form, concentration or quality that is not found in nature. Sugar comes in several forms and many disguises. The most common form is sucrose or what we know as table sugar. This is a 'dissacharide', a compound that is made up of one molecule of glucose that is linked to one molecule of fructose. So it contains 50% glucose and 50% fructose. When it is metabolised it is converted into separate molecules of glucose and fructose. These are both simple sugars or 'monosaccharides'. There is a third monosaccharide galactose. All other types of sugar are made from these three monosaccharides.

Glucose is the most important sugar as it is provides the primary source of fuel that is used throughout our body. Our body stores glucose in the liver and our muscles in the form of glycogen and this can be easily broken down back into glucose to provide energy when we need it. Galactose is the least common simple monosaccharide sugar. It is found mainly in dairy products in the form of lactose, which is one molecule of galactose linked to one molecule of glucose. In this form it is easily converted into glucose when it is metabolised. Fructose is found in fruit. Unlike galactose it cannot be converted into glucose and used throughout our body. If our body is desperately short of glucose our muscles can use it but as this rarely happens most of the fructose we consume in converted into glycogen by the liver. If the glycogen stores in the liver are full fructose is rapidly converted into fat. The fructose found in whole fruit is not bad as the rate at which it is absorbed is slowed down by the fibre the fruit contains.

Table sugar (sucrose), High Fructose Corn Syrup, Agave Nectar, Honey and Brown Rice Syrup are the five most commonly found forms of 'sugar' and they each contain different amounts of glucose and fructose.

## Table Sugar:

This is the most common form of sugar. It is often called sucrose. It contains 50% glucose and 50% fructose Although table sugar is not absorbed by the stomach it is absorbed very quickly. It is absorbed at a rate of around 30 calories a minute through the small intestine and it requires very little digestive effort. When you drink a 'regular' can of soft drink all of the sugar will be absorbed in about 5 minutes and this creates a massive sugar rush. Other food takes longer as it depends on how long it takes the food to pass through the stomach into the small intestine. As table sugar is 50% fructose half of it can be potentially stored as fat.

## High Fructose Corn Syrup:

This is a manufactured product that is made from corn. It contains 55% fructose and 45% glucose. This means that instead of 50% of the 'sugar' potentially being stored as fat as is the case when you consume table sugar or sucrose, when you consume HFCS 55% is likely to end up as fat.

From a dietary perspective this makes HFCS worse than table sugar but only by a small amount. Agreed, that 5% extra will build up and add to the pounds over time, but the real issue with HFCS is that it is cheap, much cheaper than table sugar and because of this it is used in almost all of the processed and packaged foods that we eat.

### Agave Nectar

Notwithstanding that this is presented and marketed as a healthy 'low-glycemic sweetener' Agave Nectar contains far more fructose than High Fructose Corn Syrup; it is between 85% and 90% fructose. This means that in every 10 grams it will only supply 1 gram of energy that can be used immediately. The other 9 grams will be stored either as glycogen or as fat. When you consume a 7 gram teaspoon you are effectively consuming 6 grams of fat. Because it is mainly fructose it doesn't promote the release of insulin but despite the marketing hype this is most definitely not a healthy sugar.

### Honey

Honey contains around 50% fructose, 41% glucose and 9% maltose. Maltose a disaccharide that is formed from two glucose molecules so when honey is broken down it is similar in composition to table sugar. On the positive side it does contain some trace elements and minerals but in reality this doesn't make it any healthier than normal table sugar.

### Brown Rice Syrup

This is something that has been used in the Far East for many years. Because rice is not a fruit it does not contain any fructose. Brown rice syrup is not quite as sweet as sugar and it contains 3% glucose, 45% maltose and 52% maltotriose which is a trisaccharide (i.e. three sugars) formed from three glucose molecules. Because brown rice syrup is 100% glucose, once it is broken down all of the sugar will be absorbed and used as energy. Advocates of brown rice syrup claim that the maltotriose is digested and absorbed more slowly that glucose or maltose and because of this it will sustain you for longer. While it will not be absorbed at the rate of 30 calories a minute, the energy buffer it provides is very little different to the energy buffer provided by a portion of brown rice.

So to summarise. Sugar is sugar which ever way you look at it. Irrespective of what form it comes in it gives rise to spikes in insulin levels and it contains calories. Unless you burn these calories up the excess calories will be turned into fat. The bottom line is that added sugar is of no benefit and it does not contribute to our health. It can have an adverse impact on our sensitivity to complex flavours and by altering our palette it can decrease our appreciation of other foods that are a healthy option. The best thing we can do is to train ourselves to appreciate whole unsweetened foods and to enjoy the sugars that are found naturally in whole fruits and vegetables.

## Artificial Sweeteners

In order to counter our addiction to sweet things and the excess calories they provide, over the years scientists and food technologists have developed many artificial sweeteners. These substances taste sweet but they provide fewer calories. While they satisfy our cravings for sweet things there is a lot of controversy over whether they are good for us or whether they actually cause damage.

Today there are basically four different artificial sweeteners on the market;

- Sucralose, the sweetener found in Splenda.
- Aspartame which is sold under the name of Equal and Nutrasweet and found in many 'diet' drinks.
- Saccharin, which because of a major health scare many years ago is rarely found these days.
- Stevia, the new kid on the block which is sold under various names, including Supermarket own brands.

There are other types of artificial sweeteners but they are not commonly found.

With the exception of Stevia, all of these artificial sweeteners are man made products that are not found in nature and they are all known to have side effects. Most have been linked to various levels of toxicity. Aspartame is the subject of great debate and despite many industry sponsored studies a very large question mark hangs over it.

Without getting in to the detail of the different types of artificial sweeteners and their various side effects and alleged toxicity, the main reason to avoid them is all about their purpose. At the end of the day artificial sweeteners are about reducing the number of calories we consume from sugar. But all the evidence shows that in the long term all they do is increase our daily intake of calories. Put in very simple terms artificial sweeteners confuse our brain. Because our body does not get the sweet things it is expecting, it doesn't get the 'sugar kick', the glucose 'high'. The end result is that we end up eating more. Over time the end result is that we end up eating more and we also end up eating more of the wrong things because artificial sweeteners also influence our taste in food. We begin craving more and more sugary sweet things.

Artificial sweeteners also influence our eating habits in other ways. When we consume food and drink that contains them we are less likely to make healthy choices with the other food we eat. Because we feel that we have in some way restrained ourselves and done the 'right thing', indulging ourselves a little in the other food we eat is a fairly natural response. More often than not the result of this indulgence in some unhealthy choices results in more calories than we would otherwise have consumed.

There is plenty of evidence out there that tells us that artificial sweeteners are not a good idea. They trick our brain in terms of the hormones it produces when we eat and they affect us psychologically. Their use consistently leads to increased calorie intake, not reduced calorie intake. It is an undisputed fact that the BMI of people who consume low calorie 'diet' drinks on a regular basis increases over time and overall their BMI is consistently higher than the BMI of people who do not drink regular or diet drinks.

So short of retraining our palette away from sweet to savoury what is the best artificial sweetener to use? Well the only real option is Stevia but, and its a big but, Stevia is a relatively new kid on the block that only obtained FDA approval in 2008, and this was after intensive lobbying and pressure by big business. In reality the jury is still out.

### Stevia:

Just like sugar Stevia is a natural food. It comes from the leaves of a plant that has been used by people for hundreds of years and by diabetic patients in Asia for decades. It is between 350 and 450 times sweeter than sugar. There are many claims that Stevia may actually be beneficial as it contains compounds called diterpenes that have been found to have anti-microbial, anti-fungal and antioxidant activity. Experiments have shown that it can increase insulin sensitivity, improve glucose tolerance and reduce blood glucose and it does not apparently increase appetite. Stevia is currently being research as a potential treatment for type 2 Diabetes.

The specific 'sweet' compounds in Stevia are some diterpenes that are called steviol glycosides. Because one of these compounds leaves a slightly bitter after taste, when Stevia is sold as a packaged artificial sweetener only one of the steviol glycosides is used, Rebaudioside A, as this is the sweetest compound. Like all plants and vegetables Stevia contains a number of different compounds which all work together. The laboratory experiments that have identified all of the beneficial properties of Stevia have used whole leaves of the plant dissolved in water, not just one of the steviol glycocides. There is no doubt that Rebaudioside A can claim some benefits but this could be less than the benefits from consuming the whole leaf in its natural form. Simply by extracting one glycocide Stevia has been changed, it is no longer 'natural'. It is also intensely sweet so unless it is in liquid form it needs to be 'bulked up' in order to make it usable. The bulking agent most commonly used? Maltodextrin. In other words, a highly refined carbohydrate, and this contains 4 calories per gram. How many calories in a gram of sugar? You guessed it 4!. So the whole concept behind powdered Stevia is that it has the same calories content as sugar but because it is so intensely sweet you simply use much less of it.

The solution? Try to retrain your palette and don't sweeten things at all. Failing that, the best option is to find a Stevia plant and grow it yourself and use the leaves. That way you get the full benefit of the plant. It is a tropical herb so for most of us it will not grow well outside but it will do quite well on a sunny window sill.

## Brewing Tea

Irrespective of whether it is green, white or oolong tea, making tea is all about the quality of water you use, the temperature of the water, the number of tea leaves you use and how long you leave the tea to brew for.

The basic rules are:

- The hotter the water the more bitter the tea.
- The longer the brewing time the stronger the flavour and the greater the number of flavonoids extracted.
- The more tea leaves you infuse the more flavour and the more flavonoids you extract.

Once it is taken off of the tea leaves and filtered, the longer the tea is left standing the more it will oxidise and the darker its colour will become. Depending on the type of tea, this can have a marked effect of its taste.

### Different Types of Tea

There are hundreds of different types and quality of tea; green, white, oolong and black tea and their price varies enormously. Broadly they fall into the following categories.

- Green tea: this includes green tea that is mixed with jasmine flowers and green tea leaves that are wrapped around jasmine flowers. These are called jasmine pearls
- White tea
- Oolong tea: this includes jade or green oolongs, amber oolongs and dark oolongs

Unlike conventional black tea, green, white and oolong teas can be brewed more than once so a little goes a long way.

### Water

The quality of the water you use to make the tea has a major impact on its taste. Unfiltered water has an adverse impact and it often results in a 'scum' forming on the surface of the tea. The tea will also not look bright. So if possible always try to use filtered or bottled water.

## How much tea do I use?

Clearly the more tea in the pot the potentially stronger the brew. However, the amount of tea you use really depends on the type of tea and your own personal taste. The one thing to remember is that this type of tea is drunk much weaker than conventional 'black' tea. Most Asian stores that sell tea also sell small measuring spoons and this makes the 'how much to use' a little easier. These usually hold about 2 teaspoons or 5ml. So as a rough guide, for a pot that holds two and a half pints or 1.3 litres use the following:

- basic green tea like 'gunpowder', use about a quarter of a spoon or half a teaspoon
- ordinary jasmine tea use a level spoon or 2 teaspoons
- jasmine pearls, count them out and use 40, no more
- jade oolong, a little less than one spoon, so slightly less than 2 teaspoons
- amber oolong, about three quarters of a spoon or one and a half teaspoons
- dark oolong, about half a spoon or 1 teaspoon
- the leaves of white tea are not packed tightly so for white tea use your fingers or tea tweezers.

At the end of the day it is all about personal taste, some use a simple rule of thumb of 1 gram to a litre independent of the tea being brewed.

## Water Temperature

Different types of tea need to be made with water at different temperatures. Never use boiling water. It totally destroys the flavour of the tea and it makes it very bitter. It also reduces the amount of flavonoids.

The Chinese have some interesting descriptions of the temperature of the water:-

- Shrimp eyes - 70°C/158°F – 80°C/176°F
- Crab eyes - 80°C/176°F – 85°C/185°F

- Fish eyes - 85°- C/185°F – 90°C/194°F
- Rope of Pearls - 90°C/194°F – 95°C/203°F
- Raging torrent - 95°C/203°F – 100°C/212°F
- Old man water - 100°C/212°F (over-boiled, 'flat' water)

So temperature guidelines for first brew are:

- White tea : Small shrimp eyes. May be as cool as 60ºC
- Green tea including jasmine and pearls : Shrimp eye. About 72ºC for first brew
- Oolongs : Crab / Fish eyes. 85ºC for first brew

## Brewing time

The time between adding water and filtering the tea is generally 5 minutes but can be shorter. For instance the green Japanese tea Sencha needs only about 2 minutes using 70 deg C water. The longer it is brewed for the stronger it will become and the more flavonoids will be extracted. Tea brewed for 7 minutes contains about 60% more flavonoids than tea brewed for 3 minutes.

Second and subsequent Brews.

You can use the same tea leaves 2 or 3 times. Usually hotter water is used and the tea is brewed for longer.

## Stirring and Pouring

Stirring the tea as it is brewing shortens the brewing time. It is said that pouring the tea into a glass or cup from a height so that it bubbles enhances the flavour. However, as this increases the oxidation of the tea it is maybe not such a good idea.

Last but not least you need a fine tea strainer, not the coarse ones you use for black tea. You can usually find these in the Asian supermarkets that sell tea or specialist on-line shops.

# Primers

## 1: Organic and Inorganic Compounds

Organic compounds always contain carbon and oxygen and almost all of them also contain hydrogen. The name organic relates to the historical link between these compounds and living organisms. Inorganic compounds are ones that can be derived from non living sources. Confusingly some inorganic compounds also contain carbon, carbon dioxide for example. There are far more organic compounds than inorganic compounds. So far around 7 million have been discovered.

## 2: Metabolism, Enzymes and Co-factors

### Metabolism – Part 1:

The human body is an extremely complex organism. In effect it is a massive biological engine that is fuelled by the food we eat and the air we breathe. In the cells that make up our bodies thousands of different biochemical reactions are taking place each second, converting food and oxygen into the energy we need and the materials and compounds that make up our bodies. Together these chemical reactions make up our metabolism. Food is consumed, broken down and transformed into the enormous number of different materials that our body needs; blood, muscle, skin, bone, hair, teeth. The list is very long. Most of these chemical reactions are helped along by a specific type of protein called an enzyme.

### Enzymes:

Enzymes act as catalysts. They enable a chemical reaction to take place. In fact the chemical reaction can not take place at all unless the enzyme is present, however, in the process of helping with the chemical reaction the enzyme itself is not changed. Enzymes are able to catalyse thousands of reactions at the same time. They are extremely efficient. The body contains thousands of different enzymes and each of these is finely tuned to undertake a specific task. Some enzymes are able to act as a catalyst on their own. Others, called apoenzymes, require a small molecule known as a co-factor to assist with the catalysing activity. In other words, they are inactive and only become active when a co-factor is present.

### Co-factors and Co-enzymes:

A co-factor is a non protein molecule that binds to an enzyme and enables the enzyme to become active. Co-factors can be either co-enzymes or inorganic molecules in the form of metal ions. Co-enzymes are small organic molecules that are often derived from vitamins.

### Metabolic Pathways:

When our bodies transform a food molecule into a different molecule it does this in a sequence of steps. Each of these steps is catalysed by a specific enzyme. The sequence of steps and the series of enzymes that take part in the conversion of one molecule into another is its metabolic pathway. There are thousands of metabolic pathways in our bodies.

### Metabolism – Part 2:

Metabolism is divided into two different processes, Catabolism and Anabolism.

- Catabolism - is a series of processes that breakdown large molecules of organic matter into smaller molecules that can be used to provide energy and the components needed for the body's anabolic processes. These large molecules of organic matter include proteins, sugars and fats.
- Anabolism - uses the energy and molecules broken down by catabolic processes to make the compounds needed by our bodies.

The various metabolic pathways need a constant supply of organic and inorganic compounds. Some like sodium and potassium are abundant while others work in minute concentrations. About 99% of our body mass is made up of the elements carbon, nitrogen, calcium, sodium, chlorine, potassium, hydrogen, phosphorus, oxygen and sulphur. Organic compounds in the form of carbohydrates, fats and proteins contain the majority of the carbon and nitrogen. Most of the oxygen and hydrogen is in the form of water.

## 3: Carbohydrates, Proteins and Amino Acids

### Carbohydrates:

Carbohydrates are the most abundant biological molecules and they fulfil numerous roles. The food we eat supplies us with carbohydrates in two different forms, starch and sugar. Both of these contain fibre or cellulose. Starches and sugars provide us with energy. Fibre or cellulose provides us with the 'bulk' our digestive systems need to work efficiently. With the exception of fructose all carbohydrates, irrespective of whether they are starch or sugar, are digested or metabolised to form glucose, a simple form of sugar. The body uses glucose as a source of fuel from which it generates energy.

### Proteins:

Proteins are the main tissue builders in our body. They exist in every cell and they are essential for all of the body's functions. Many proteins are the enzymes that act as the catalysts for the biochemical reactions that take place in metabolism. They also play an important part in our body's immune response. Proteins are made from amino acids. There are around twenty groups of amino acids and of these eight are essential amino acids as our bodies simply will not work without them.

### Amino Acids:

Amino acids are organic compounds that are made mainly, but not exclusively, from the elements carbon, hydrogen, oxygen and nitrogen. About 500 different amino acids are known and they are classified into different groups. In the form of proteins they comprise the second largest component after water in human muscle, cells and tissues.

## 4: Fats, Lipids and Polyunsaturated Fatty Acids

Lipid is the medical term for fat. It is a term that is usually used to refer to the fats that are found in our blood. Lipids and fats are the most diverse group of biochemicals in our body. They are regarded as the third food group after carbohydrates and proteins. Lipids and fats are a class of organic compound that are sometimes referred to as 'Fatty acids'. Lipids or fatty acids fulfil an essential role in our bodies by forming and maintaining the structure or 'casing' around our cells. They also provide a concentrated source of 'reserve' energy. On a weight for weight basis they provide twice as much energy as carbohydrates and proteins. One gram of fat yields around 9 kcals of energy whereas one gram of carbohydrate yields only 4 kcals. So our body's fat reserves contain a lot of energy and provided we have sufficient water, they can sustain a human body for many days.

There are three different groups of lipids in the body, Triglycerides, Phospholipids and Sterols or Steroids. The Triglycerides are the commonest. They perform an important role that enables fat to be both stored and then retrieved and used as a source of energy. In cells phospholipids occur with proteins and cholesterol in the membrane layer that encases the cell. Sterols are not strictly speaking fatty acids but they are considered to be a lipid because they are similar to Triglycerides and share some of the same pathways when they are made. Our sex hormones are steroid based and vitamin D is a steroid based vitamin.

## Cholesterol:

One of the fats in our bodies that we have all heard about is cholesterol. This is the principle compound in the Sterol group and it plays an important role in metabolism. About 75% of the cholesterol we need is made by our liver, the rest is obtained from our food. When we consume cholesterol in food our body regulates its own production. Because of this the intake of cholesterol from food has only a small effect on the total amount of cholesterol in our body. Cholesterol is also recycled, typically 50% of the cholesterol excreted each day is reabsorbed.

In order to travel around our body cholesterol combines with a protein to form something called a lipoprotein ( lipid + protein). This protein 'coats' the cholesterol. There are two kinds of lipoproteins, low density lipoprotein (LDL) and high density lipoprotein (HDL). LDL makes up the majority of the the cholesterol in our body. Not all cholesterol is created equal though. The HDL lipoprotein has more protein than cholesterol and it moves quickly and efficiently around our body, sometimes mopping up LDL on the way. The LDL lipoproteins however have more cholesterol than protein. They move more slowly, knocking into things and getting themselves attached to cells and the lining of our arteries. Because of this LDL's are known as 'bad cholesterol' as they can damage cells and build up in our arteries, ultimately leading to disease.

## Essential Fatty Acids:

Our bodies are able to make most of the different types of fats and fatty acids that it needs from the food we eat. However some can only be obtained directly from food. Because our bodies are unable to make them these fats are called Essential Fatty Acids or EFA's. Most of us have heard about essential fatty acids, the names Omega-3 and Omega-6 usually come to mind. There is also an Omega-9 by the way but we don't very often hear about this.

In total there are four 'groups' of polyunsaturated fatty acids; Omega-3, Omega-6, Omega-9 and Conjugated Fatty Acid and each 'group' contains a number of different types of fatty acid. Alpha Linolenic Acid (ALA) and Linoleic Acid (LA) are the two EFA's that are of interest as they are the 'parents' so to speak of the different Omega-3 and Omega- 6 groups of fatty acids that our bodies make from them.

Alpha Linolenic Acid (ALA) is the parent of the Omega-3 group and it is converted by the body into eicosapentaenoic acid (EPA) and decosahexaenoic acid (DHA). Unfortunately this conversion process is not very efficient and some scientists believe that as little as 1% of the ALA we consume ends up as DHA or EPA and this 1% conversion decreases even more with age. Luckily both DHA and EPA can be obtained directly from our food so we need to obtain a lot of DHA and EPA as well as ALA from our diet. Sadly the modern Western Diet does not provide a very good source of any of these.

Linoleic Acid (LA) is the parent of the Omega-6 group and it is converted by our bodies into Gamma-Linolenic acid (GLA) and Arachidonic Acid (AA). Unlike ALA it is readily converted into GLA and AA and our Western Diet provides an abundant source of Linoleic Acid.

As well as playing several crucial roles in our body EPA and DHA have powerful anti-inflammatory properties. GLA and AA have powerful pro-inflammatory properties. Our Western Diet which is high in polyunsaturated vegetable oils provides an abundant source of Linoleic Acid. This means that we end up with an imbalance in the ratio of Omega 3 and Omega 6 and this can gear up the inflammation process.

## 5: Vitamins and Minerals

### Vitamins:

Vitamins were first identified in 1905 by a British doctor named William Fletcher who was researching the causes of a tropical disease called Beriberi. In 1906 a biochemist named Frederick Gowland Hopkins discovered that certain nutritional parts of food were important to health. It wasn't until 1911 that a Polish scientist called Cashmir Funk named these special nutritional parts of food as a vitamine - 'vita' meaning life and 'amine' from a compound called Thiamine that he had been studying. Over the years the vitamins as we know them today were discovered.

Vitamin C is probably the one vitamin we are all aware of and it has an interesting history. In 1747 a Scottish naval surgeon James Lind discovered that something in citrus fruit prevented scurvy. As a consequence a few years after this British sailors were given lime juice as part of their daily rations - hence their nickname 'Limeys'. The information about the nutritional content of citrus fruit was lost but then rediscovered by two Norwegians in 1912. Vitamin C was the first vitamin to be artificially made in 1935.

Vitamins are organic compounds. Although they are only needed in small quantities they are essential for the body to function correctly. Deficiencies in any of the essential vitamins can cause health problems. Likewise, research now suggests that an excess of certain vitamins, especially when they are taken in the form of supplements, can also cause health problems. Because our bodies are unable to make vitamins they need to come from our food. A large number of vitamins are essential but some are more important than others. As is the case with Vitamin C without it sailors became ill with scurvy and ultimately they died.

There are 13 essential vitamins and these are divided into two groups, fat soluble vitamins and water soluble vitamins: The 4 fat soluble vitamins are stored in the body's fatty tissues; these are vitamins A, D, E and K. The body is unable to store the 9 water soluble vitamins; these are the B group of vitamins - B1 thiamine, B2 riboflavin, B3 niacin, B5 pantothenic acid, B6 pyridoxine, B7 biotin, B9 folic acid and B12 cobolamin. The 9th water soluble vitamin is Vitamin C. All of these water soluble vitamins need to be used straight away and replaced each day. With the exception of vitamin B12 which can be stored in the liver for many years, any of the water soluble vitamins that are not used are excreted.

### Minerals.

While minerals do not contribute directly to our energy needs they play an important part as 'regulators' of some of our body's functions. They also play a role in some metabolic pathways where they work with enzymes as co-factors. More than fifty minerals are found in the body and about twenty-five of these are thought to be essential. Nutritionists classify minerals as being either macro minerals or trace elements. The body stores varying amounts of minerals but it needs to maintain a steady supply in order to make up for losses.

## 6: Insulin, Leptin and Ghrelin

Insulin, Leptin and Ghrelin are three hormones that have a major influence on our bodies. They work together and allow our bodies to process the food we eat and recognise and respond to feelings of hunger, fullness (satiety) and our overall state of nutrition. Ghrelin is the 'hunger hormone' and Leptin is the 'full' or 'satiety' hormone.

The pancreas produces a hormone called insulin when we consume any type of carbohydrate; bread, cereals, pasta, vegetables, cakes, sugar and sweetened drinks all contain carbohydrates. Once consumed all carbohydrates are eventually broken down into glucose and used throughout our body as the 'fuel' it needs to generate energy. As food is metabolised and the level of glucose in the blood increases insulin is released. Insulin has the job of regulating the amount of glucose that is circulating in our blood by telling it to store the glucose that is not immediately needed in muscle cells and in the liver in the form of glycogen. The insulin causes a reduction in the release of Ghrelin, the hunger hormone, and an increase in the release of Leptin, the satiety hormone, which signals to your brain that you have eaten enough food. The Leptin in turn reduces the amount of insulin that the body produces.

When food is in short supply the overall amount of carbohydrates that you consume reduces. This results in a drop in insulin levels because insulin is released in direct response to the amount of carbohydrates you eat. The low insulin levels cause a rise in Ghrelin which makes you feel hungry, so you go and find food to eat. The low insulin also stimulates Leptin to breakdown and release stored fat from fat cells so that it can be used as energy. As these fat cells shrink in size they produce less Leptin. The lower Leptin levels mean that your metabolic rate falls and as a consequence you burn up calories more slowly, protecting yourself from food shortage. So what happens when we consume too many calories?

## Insulin Resistance

Insulin levels rise in line with glucose levels but the muscle cells and the liver become full. The full cells become less responsive to insulin and they become resistant to it so your blood sugar spikes. The pancreas produces even more insulin in an attempt to reduce the high level of glucose in the blood. The high level of insulin prevents the release of fat from your fat cells so you are not burning any body fat. Eventually, as the fat cells are resistant and muscle cells are resistant and probably full, the glucose has no where to go but to the liver for conversion into glycogen. The liver fills up quickly, so the extra glucose is converted into fatty acids in the form of lipoproteins. These lipoproteins are then ushered into fat tissue for conversion into triglycerides which are stored as body fat. If you lead a fairly sedentary life your body does not consume much energy so your glycogen stores usually stay full, so more carbohydrates means more glucose and this has no where to go but into fat cells.

The result is insulin resistance and the development of higher and higher insulin levels which drives the process forward even more. Too much carbohydrate and lack of exercise create a vicious circle where Leptin, Ghrelin and insulin combine to add on those extra pounds and cause insulin resistance and ultimately metabolic syndrome.

## 7: Metabolic Syndrome

Sometimes referred to as Syndrome X, Metabolic Syndrome is regarded by many as a worldwide epidemic. It is estimated that 1 in 4 adults in the UK suffer from it and 1 in 3 of the American adult population meet the criteria for Metabolic Syndrome set down by National Institutes of Health.

Metabolic Syndrome is a medical term used to describe a combination of insulin resistance, diabetes, high blood pressure and obesity. It puts you at greater risk of heart disease, stroke and other conditions affecting blood vessels. People with Metabolic Syndrome are overweight, have high levels of triglycerides and low levels of good HDL cholesterol, high blood pressure, Insulin Resistance and a tendency to develop inflammation.

## 8: Glycemic Index

The Glycemic Index (GI) is a way of ranking foods that contain carbohydrates based on their effect on blood glucose levels. The change in blood glucose levels following a meal is determined by the relative amount and availability of the carbohydrates to digestive enzymes and the presence of dietary factors such as fat and fibre which slows down the rate at which carbohydrates are digested. Different cooking methods can also reduce or increase the rate at which carbohydrate foods are digested. Foods that are absorbed slowly have a low GI rating, while foods that are absorbed more quickly have a higher GI rating. Choosing carbohydrates that are slowly absorbed instead of carbohydrates that are quickly absorbed can help even out blood glucose levels. Complex carbohydrates will almost always have a lower Glycemic Index than refined carbohydrates.

Foods are given a GI number according to their effect on blood glucose levels. Glucose is used as the standard reference (GI 100) and other foods are measured against this. The effect on blood glucose levels of a portion of food containing say 50g of carbohydrate over a three hour period is compared to the effect of 50g of glucose over the same period.

- Low GI foods have a glycemic index of 55 or less
- Medium GI foods have a glycemic index of between 56 and 69
- High GI foods have a glycemic index of 70 or above

Determining the glycemic index of a meal is not as easy as reading a number off of a chart because various factors can affect the glycemic index of a food:

- Cooking methods: frying, boiling and baking: For example potatoes that are sautéed have a lower GI than potatoes that are boiled or microwaved. This is because sautéing is less destructive to the starchy potato carbohydrates than boiling and as a consequence they are digested more slowly.
- Processing and the ripeness of fruit and certain vegetables affects their glycemic index. The riper the fruit the higher its GI.
- Whole grains and high fibre foods act as a physical barrier that slows down the digestion and absorption of carbohydrate. So adding pulses to rice reduces its GI
- Fat lowers the GI of a food. For example chocolate has a medium GI because of its fat content, so adding fat to a high GI food will reduce its glycemic index.
- Protein lowers the GI of food. Milk and other dairy products have a low GI because of their high protein content, and because they also contain fat.
- Foods that are slightly acidic slow down the rate at which the stomach empties and this slows their rate of digestion. So adding lemon juice or vinegar to carbohydrate foods has the effect of lowering their GI. As an example, sour dough bread has a lower GI than standard bread.

Another index that is used when measuring the nutritional content of food is its 'Glycemic Load' or GL. This takes into account the Glycemic Index (GI) of the food and the amount of carbohydrate in a portion of the food; think about a slice of melon and a slice of white bead. You can also change the overall glycemic load by combining different foods. The glycemic load gives you a more accurate picture of what really happens when you eat carbohydrates.

Low GI foods that release their carbohydrates slowly reduce the peaks in blood glucose levels that follow a meal. Although research findings vary, most agree that there appears to be a favourable effect on good HDL cholesterol after the consumption of a low GI diet. There is also some evidence that consuming lower GI foods reduces the inflammatory response.

## 9: Saturated Solutions and Crystallisation

Crystallisation happens when solid crystals are formed or precipitate out of a solution. It is essentially a solid to liquid separation technique that separates a chemical from the solvent in which is is dissolved. Crystals can form in different shapes and sizes. Usually in order for crystallisation to take place a solution needs to be 'supersaturated'. This refers to a state in which the liquid or solvent contains more dissolved solids than it can hold at a given temperature. As the temperature drops crystals begin to form. However, the first step in crystallisation is a process called nucleation. Usually some form of force, a change in temperature or a small particle that 'seeds' the nucleation process is needed for this to happen.

## 10: pH and Acidosis

Power of Hydrogen pH, sometimes called Potential of Hydrogen, is a measure of the acidity or alkalinity of a solution. It measures the balance between positively charged ions that are acid forming and negatively charged ions that are alkaline forming. pH is measured on a scale of 0 to 14, the lower the pH the more acidic the solution, the higher the pH the more alkaline (or base) the solution. When a solution is neither acid or alkaline it has a pH of 7 which is neutral. Pure water is generally considered to have a neutral pH of 7. It is important to note that on the pH scale, each number represents a ten fold difference from the adjacent number; in other words a liquid that has a pH of 6 is ten times more acidic than pure water that has a pH of 7, a liquid with a pH of 5 is one hundred times more acidic than pure water.

Water is the most abundant compound in our body. In fact about 70% of our body is water. The body has an acid to alkaline, (or acid to base) ratio of between 7.35 and 7.45, so it is slightly more alkaline than pure water. If the pH of your blood falls below 7.35 the result is a condition called acidosis. If it rises above 7.45 the result is alkalosis. The pH of our blood is tightly regulated by a complex system of buffers that are continuously at work striving on a moment to moment basis to balance our pH. When this balance is severely compromised many medical problems can occur.

So is it true that the food and drink we consume causes our blood to become more alkaline or acidic?

Well contrary to what we are led to believe, not to any significant degree. As part of our everyday metabolic activity our cells are continuously producing energy and in the process of doing this a number of different acids are formed and released into our body fluids. When we consume food and drink the end products of digestion and the assimilation of nutrients often results in an acid or alkaline forming effect. Fortunately our body has three major mechanisms that work constantly to prevent dietary, metabolic and other factors from pushing the pH of our blood outside of the 7.35 to 7.45 range. When people encourage you to 'alkalise your blood' most of them mean that you should eat plenty of foods that have an overall alkaline forming effect. The reason for making this suggestion is that the vast majority of highly processed foods, like white flour and white sugar have an acid forming effect and if you spend years eating a poor diet that is mainly acid forming you will over work some of your body's buffering systems to a point where you could create undesirable changes in your health.

## Potential Renal Acid Load

When reading about foods that have an acid forming effect you may have read about their PRAL index. This stands for Potential Renal Acid Load, a method of determining the level of the food's acidity. However, foods can be misleading as they can contain acid, for example tomatoes, but when they are digested and metabolised they have an alkaline effect on the body.

## 11: The Redox cycle

Redox is short for REDuction and OXidation reactions that take place in our body. REDOX reactions are usually associated with a gain or loss of electrons, but there are some REDOX reactions that do not involve the transfer of electrons. Depending on the chemical reaction, reduction and oxidation may involve any of the following for a given atom, ion or molecule:

- Reduction involves the gain of electrons or hydrogen OR the loss of oxygen OR a decease in oxidation state.
- Oxidation involves the loss of electrons or hydrogen OR the gain of oxygen OR an increase in oxidation state.

There is no net change of charge in a REDOX reaction, so the excess electrons in the oxidation reaction must equal the number of electrons consumed by the reduction reaction. Redox reactions are a vital part of the chemical reactions that take place in our bodies. The electron transfer system in our cells and the oxidation of glucose in our body are examples of them.

## 12: Free Radicals and Antioxidants

### Free Radicals:

A Free Radical is an atom, molecule or compound that is highly unstable because of its atomic or molecular structure. Any molecule or atom that has one or more unpaired or 'free' electrons in its outer orbit is known as a Free Radical. Free radicals attempt to stabilise themselves by reacting with other atoms, molecules or even individual electrons to create a stable compound. In order to do this they 'steal' an electron from another atom or molecule, bind to another molecule or interact in various ways with other Free Radicals.

Reactive Oxygen Species, ROS, is a collective term used to describe all of the Free Radicals commonly found in biology. It includes not only oxygen based free radicals but also some derivatives of oxygen such as hydrogen peroxide, singlet oxygen (superoxide), peroxynitrite and hypochlorous acid that are not technically free radicals. A similar term is used to describe free radicals that are derived from nitrogen, Reactive

Nitrogen Species or RNS.

The majority of life forms that exist on earth need oxygen to live, yet one of the paradoxes of this is that oxygen is a highly reactive molecule that can damage living organisms by producing free radicals and Reactive Oxygen Species. Simply by living and deriving energy from the air we breathe and the food we eat our bodies produce Free Radicals. Many of these are needed in controlled amounts to maintain life and keep us in good health, others however can react with cells, fats and proteins inside our bodies and cause damage. Free radicals and Reactive Oxygen Species are all around us. We breath them in from cigarette smoke, car exhausts and air pollution, the ultra violet rays from the sun create them when we are exposed to sunlight and we consume them in our food and sometimes the water we drink.

An imbalance or overload of Free Radicals can impair the immune system and it is a potential factor in many modern day illnesses. In order for us to be able to lead healthy lives the Reactive Oxygen Species and Free Radicals need to be neutralised and rendered harmless. In order to do this we need antioxidants.

## Antioxidants:

The word antioxidants refers to any molecule that is capable of stabilising or deactivating free radicals. Antioxidants are stable molecules that have electrons to spare. When antioxidants come into contact with free radicals and Reactive Oxygen Species they hand over their electrons and neutralise the free radicals by binding to them and effectively 'making them safe'. The human body has a complex internally produced defence against free radicals, a sophisticated armoury of antioxidants that is uses to defend and protect itself by inhibiting free radical formation, neutralising free radicals that are already formed and repairing any oxidative damage that has occurred. In addition, antioxidants are contained in the food we eat; Vitamin C (ascorbate), Vitamin E and the beta carotenes are just some of the 8,000 antioxidants that nature provides us with. Some antioxidants work as a team or network as they can interact with other antioxidants to regenerate their original properties once they have been used.

When our antioxidant defences are over powered by Free Radicals and when free radicals increase at a rate that is faster than our body's ability to increase its own antioxidant defences, the disturbance in the antioxidant to pro-oxidant balance shifts in favour of the free radicals and damage to the body and Oxidative Stress occurs.

### Lipid Peroxidation:

This happens when free radicals disrupt the fats and fatty membranes that are around and inside cells. It is a process that damages cells and can ultimately lead to the death of cells. One of the main functions of Vitamin E is to protect against lipid peroxidation.

## 13: Oxidative stress

Oxidative Stress exists when there is an imbalance between free radicals and the body's ability to render them harmless or repair the damage they have caused. The body either has an inadequate supply of antioxidants or it is creating or being exposed to too many free radicals. When this happens the free radicals and ROS oxidise and damage cells and other components of the cells such as fats (lipids), proteins, and nucleic acids (DNA and RNA). This leads to the influx of inflammatory cells to the sites of the injury and on some occassions cells die. The effect of Oxidative Stress depends on the size or scale of the imbalance between the free radicals and the antioxidants. A cell is able to overcome small amounts of damage and regain its original state, but more severe Oxidative Stress can have toxic effects that can result in widespread cell death.

## 14: Inflammation

Inflammation is a topic that is attracting a lot of attention at the moment as it appears to be connected to many chronic diseases. The word inflammation comes from the Latin word 'inflammo' meaning 'I set alight, I ignite'. When something harmful or irritating affects a part of your body there is an automatic biological response to try to remove it. When you catch a cold or sprain your ankle your immune system moves into gear and triggers a chain of events called the inflammatory cascade. The familiar signs of inflammation, raised temperature, localised heat, pain, swelling and redness, are the first signs that your immune system is being called into action and they show that the body is trying to heal itself.

Inflammation is part of the body's innate immune response, something that is present from the moment we are born. Innate immunity is an automatic non specific immunity but as we go through life we acquire adaptive immunity as we are exposed to diseases or vaccinated against them. In a delicate balance of give-and-take inflammation begins when 'pro-inflammatory hormones' in your body call out for your white blood cells to come and clear out infection or repair damaged tissue. These pro-inflammatory hormones are matched by equally powerful closely related 'anti-inflammatory' compounds which move in once the threat is neutralised to begin the healing process.

The inflammation we experience during our daily lives can be either 'acute' or 'chronic'. Chronic inflammation is sometimes referred to as 'systemic' inflammation.

Acute inflammation that ebbs and flows as needed signifies a well balanced immune system. Colds, flu and childhood diseases mean that inflammation and a rise in temperature starts suddenly and quickly progresses to become severe. The signs and symptoms are only present for a few days and they soon subside. In cases of severe illness they can last for a few weeks.

Sometimes however, as in the case of chronic or systemic inflammation, the inflammation itself can cause further inflammation. It can become self perpetuating and sometimes last for months or even years. Symptoms of inflammation that don't go away are telling you that the 'on' switch to your immune system is stuck. It's poised on high alert and won't shut off. Some people believe that chronic irritants, food sensitivities and common allergens like proteins found in dairy products and wheat can trigger this type of chronic inflammation.

There is no doubt that in the western world chronic or systemic inflammation is on the rise. We know this from inflammatory markers and the pro-inflammatory and anti-inflammatory hormones that our body produces. One of these, C-Reactive Protein, (CRP) is a protein that binds to dead and dying cells and bacteria in order to clear them out from the body. It can always be found and measured in the blood stream, but levels of CRP spike when there is inflammation. CRP is highly sensitive and its levels increase rapidly in response to any type of inflammation. CRP tells us that inflammation is present but it doesn't tell us what is causing the inflammation.

Interleukin-6 (IL-6) is another inflammatory maker that is secreted by two different types of cells; white blood cells called a T-cells, and macrophages. The macrophages are the cells that engulf and digest stray tissue and pathogens. T-cells and macrophages play a huge role in our immune response. Systemic inflammation does not result in the sweeping response of trauma but it keeps the body in a constant state of being 'in repair' mode. Immune cells like the macrophages take charge and a recurring destructive process of tissue destruction and repair takes over.

Without getting into the biochemistry in too much detail, there is a complicated interaction between inflammatory messengers, cytokines, prostaglandins and the short lived hormones inside our cells called eicosanoids which can act as either pro-inflammatory and anti-inflammatory compounds. Put simply, the anti-inflammatory eicosanoids draw upon the Omega-3 fatty acids in our tissues and the pro-inflammatory eicosanoids draw on the Omega-6 fatty acids. In order to maintain a proper inflammatory response we need both of these eicosanoids but with high levels of Omega-6 we end up making far too many pro-inflammatory eicosanoids and not enough anti-inflammatory ones.

Prostaglandins are a sort of chemical messenger. They are made from Arachiodonic Acid (AA) by two different enzymes, COX-1 and COX-2. Prostaglandins have slightly different effects on the body that depend on which enzyme was used when they were made. The COX-1 enzyme is always present but the COX-2 enzyme is not usually detectable in normal tissue, it only becomes abundant at sites of inflammation.

If you suffer from gout you will have heard of NSAID's, Non Steroidal Anti-inflammatory Drugs. These work by blocking the COX-1 and COX-2 enzymes and preventing them catalysing the formation of inflammatory prostaglandins from Arachiodonic Acid. Omega-3 fatty acids work in the same way and the EPA that is derived from them also acts as a COX inhibitor.

## 15: How Purines Become Uric Acid

The following is included to illustrate how the purines Guanine and Adenine are converted to uric acid and how other purines are 'salvaged' in the process:

The purine Guanine:

- A nuclease frees the nucleotide
- A nucleotidase creates guanosine
- Purine nucleoside phosphorylase converts guanoise to guanine
- Guanase converts guanine to xanthine
- Xanthine oxidase ( a form of xanthine oxidoreductase) catalyses the oxidation of xanthine to uric acid

The purine Adenine:

- A nuclease frees the nucleotide
- A nucleotidase creates adenosine then adenosine deaminase creates inosine
- Alternatively, AMP deaminase creates inosinic acid then a nucleotidase creates insoine
- Purine nucleoside phosphorylase acts upon inosine to create hypoxanthineXanthine oxidoreductase catalyses the bio transformation of hypoxanthine to xanthine
- Xanthine oxidoreductase acts upon xanthine to create uric acid

Purines from the turnover of nucleic acids and from food can also be salvaged and reused in new nucleotides.

- The enzyme adenine phosphoribosyltransferase (APT) salvages adenine
- The enzyme hypoxanthine-guanine phosphoribosyl transferase (HGPRT) salvages guanine and hypoxanthine

# Recipe Index

# List of Recipes

# Index

CPSIA information can be obtained
at www.ICGtesting.com
Printed in the USA
BVHW061258260122
627131BV00014B/543

9 781999 624811